# Crisis Standards of Care

## SUMMARY OF A WORKSHOP SERIES

Clare Stroud, Bruce M. Altevogt, Lori Nadig, and
Matthew Hougan, *Rapporteurs*

Forum on Medical and Public Health
for Catastrophic Even

Board on Health Sciences Policy

### INSTITUTE OF MEDICINE
OF THE NATIONAL ACADEMIES

THE NATIONAL ACADEMIES PRESS
Washington, D.C.
www.nap.edu

**THE NATIONAL ACADEMIES PRESS** • 500 Fifth Street, N.W. • Washington, DC 20001

NOTICE: The project that is the subject of this report was approved by the Governing Board of the National Research Council, whose members are drawn from the councils of the National Academy of Sciences, the National Academy of Engineering, and the Institute of Medicine. The members of the committee responsible for the report were chosen for their special competences and with regard for appropriate balance.

This project was supported by contracts between the National Academy of Sciences and the American College of Emergency Physicians, the American Hospital Association, the American Medical Association, the American Nurses Association, the Association of State and Territorial Health Officials, the Centers for Disease Control and Prevention (Contract No. 200-2005-13434 TO #6), the Department of the Army (Contract No. W81XWH-08-P-0934), the Department of Health and Human Services' Agency for Healthcare Research and Quality (Contract No. HHSP233200800498P), the Department of Health and Human Services' National Institutes of Health (Contract No. N01-OD-4-2139 TO #198), the Department of Health and Human Services' Office of the Assistant Secretary for Preparedness and Response (Contract No. HHSP233200900680P), the Department of Homeland Security's Federal Emergency Management Agency (Contract No. HSFEHQ-08-P-1800), the Department of Homeland Security's Office of Health Affairs (Contract No. HSHQDC-07-C-00097), the Department of Veteran Affairs (Contract No. V101(93)P-2136 TO #10), the Emergency Nurses Association, the National Association of Chain Drug Stores, the National Association of County and City Health Officials, the National Association of Emergency Medical Technicians, the Pharmaceutical Research and Manufacturers of America, the Robert Wood Johnson Foundation, and the United Health Foundation. The views presented in this publication are those of the editors and attributing authors and do not necessarily reflect the view of the organizations or agencies that provided support for this project.

International Standard Book Number-13: 978-0-309-12666-3
International Standard Book Number-10: 0-309-12666-5

Additional copies of this report are available from The National Academies Press, 500 Fifth Street, N.W., Lockbox 285, Washington, DC 20055; (800) 624-6242 or (202) 334-3313 (in the Washington metropolitan area); Internet, http://www.nap.edu.

For more information about the Institute of Medicine, visit the IOM home page at: **www.iom.edu.**

Printed in the United States of America

Suggested citation: IOM (Institute of Medicine). 2010. *Crisis standards of care: Summary of a workshop series.* Washington, DC: The National Academies Press.

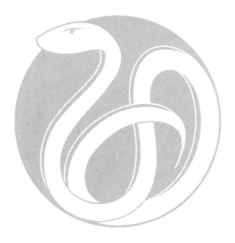

# INSTITUTE OF MEDICINE
## OF THE NATIONAL ACADEMIES

**Advising the Nation. Improving Health.**

# THE NATIONAL ACADEMIES
*Advisers to the Nation on Science, Engineering, and Medicine*

The **National Academy of Sciences** is a private, nonprofit, self-perpetuating society of distinguished scholars engaged in scientific and engineering research, dedicated to the furtherance of science and technology and to their use for the general welfare. Upon the authority of the charter granted to it by the Congress in 1863, the Academy has a mandate that requires it to advise the federal government on scientific and technical matters. Dr. Ralph J. Cicerone is president of the National Academy of Sciences.

The **National Academy of Engineering** was established in 1964, under the charter of the National Academy of Sciences, as a parallel organization of outstanding engineers. It is autonomous in its administration and in the selection of its members, sharing with the National Academy of Sciences the responsibility for advising the federal government. The National Academy of Engineering also sponsors engineering programs aimed at meeting national needs, encourages education and research, and recognizes the superior achievements of engineers. Dr. Charles M. Vest is president of the National Academy of Engineering.

The **Institute of Medicine** was established in 1970 by the National Academy of Sciences to secure the services of eminent members of appropriate professions in the examination of policy matters pertaining to the health of the public. The Institute acts under the responsibility given to the National Academy of Sciences by its congressional charter to be an adviser to the federal government and, upon its own initiative, to identify issues of medical care, research, and education. Dr. Harvey V. Fineberg is president of the Institute of Medicine.

The **National Research Council** was organized by the National Academy of Sciences in 1916 to associate the broad community of science and technology with the Academy's purposes of furthering knowledge and advising the federal government. Functioning in accordance with general policies determined by the Academy, the Council has become the principal operating agency of both the National Academy of Sciences and the National Academy of Engineering in providing services to the government, the public, and the scientific and engineering communities. The Council is administered jointly by both Academies and the Institute of Medicine. Dr. Ralph J. Cicerone and Dr. Charles M. Vest are chair and vice chair, respectively, of the National Research Council.

# Workshop Planning Committee[*]

**SALLY PHILLIPS** (*Chair*), Agency for Healthcare Research and Quality, Rockville, MD
**JAMES BLUMENSTOCK,** Association of State and Territorial Health Officials, Arlington, VA
**KATIE BREWER,** American Nurses Association, Silver Spring, MD
**KATHRYN BRINSFIELD,** Department of Homeland Security, Washington, DC
**STEPHEN CANTRILL,** Denver Health Medical Center, Denver, CO
**CAPT D. W. CHEN,** Department of Defense, Washington, DC
**JEFFREY DUCHIN,** Seattle & King County and University of Washington, Seattle, WA
**EDWARD GABRIEL,** The Walt Disney Company, Burbank, CA
**LTC(P) WAYNE HACHEY,** Department of Defense, Washington, DC
**DAN HANFLING,** Inova Health System, Falls Church, VA
**JACK HERRMANN,** National Association of County and City Health Officials, Washington, DC
**JOHN L. HICK,** Hennepin County Medical Center, Minneapolis, MN
**RADM ANN R. KNEBEL,** Department of Health and Human Services, Washington, DC
**CAPT DEBORAH LEVY,** Centers for Disease Control and Prevention, Atlanta, GA
**ANTHONY MACINTYRE,** George Washington University, Washington, DC
**MARGARET M. McMAHON,** Emergency Nurses Association, Williamstown, NJ
**CHERYL A. PETERSON,** American Nurses Association, Silver Spring, MD
**TIA POWELL,** Montefiore-Einstein Center for Bioethics, Bronx, NY
**CHERYL STARLING,** California Department of Public Health, Sacramento, CA
**ERIC TONER,** University of Pittsburgh Medical Center, Pittsburgh, PA

---

[*]IOM planning committees are solely responsible for organizing the workshop, identifying topics, and choosing speakers. The responsibility for the published workshop summary rests with the workshop rapporteurs and the institution.

*IOM Staff*

**BRUCE ALTEVOGT,** Forum Director
**CLARE STROUD,** Program Officer
**ANDREW POPE,** Director, Board on Health Sciences Policy
**MARNINA KAMMERSELL,** Research Associate
**ALEX REPACE,** Senior Program Assistant

# Forum on Medical and Public Health Preparedness for Catastrophic Events*

**LEWIS GOLDFRANK** (*Chair*), New York University Medical Center, New York, NY

**DAMON ARNOLD,** Association of State and Territorial Health Officials, Arlington, VA

**GEORGES BENJAMIN,** American Public Health Association, Washington, DC

**ROBERT DARLING,** Uniformed Services University, Bethesda, MD

**VICTORIA DAVEY,** Department of Veterans Affairs, Washington, DC

**JEFFREY DUCHIN,** Seattle & King County and University of Washington, Seattle, WA

**ELLEN EMBREY,** Office of Assistant Secretary of Defense for Health Affairs, Department of Defense, Washington, DC

**LYNN GOLDMAN,** Johns Hopkins Bloomberg School of Public Health, Baltimore, MD

**DAVID HENRY,** National Governors Association, Washington, DC

**JACK HERRMANN,** National Association of County and City Health Officials, Washington, DC

**KEITH HOLTERMANN,** Federal Emergency Management Agency, Washington, DC

**JAMES JAMES,** American Medical Association, Chicago, IL

**JERRY JOHNSTON,** National Association of Emergency Medical Technicians, Mt. Pleasant, IA

**ROBERT KADLEC,** PRTM Management Consultants, Washington, DC

**BRIAN KAMOIE,** The White House, Washington, DC

**LYNNE KIDDER,** Business Executives for National Security, Washington, DC

**JON KROHMER,** Department of Homeland Security, Washington, DC

**MICHAEL KURILLA,** National Institute of Allergy and Infectious Diseases, Bethesda, MD

---

*IOM forums and roundtables do not issue, review, or approve individual documents. The responsibility for the published workshop summary rests with the workshop rapporteurs and the institution.

JAYNE LUX, National Business Group on Health, Washington, DC
ANTHONY MACINTYRE, American College of Emergency
   Physicians, Washington, DC
ANGELA McGOWAN, Robert Wood Johnson Foundation, Princeton,
   NJ
MARGARET McMAHON, Emergency Nurses Association,
   Williamstown, NJ
ERIN MULLEN, Pharmaceutical Research and Manufacturers of
   America, Washington, DC
GERALD PARKER, Office of the Assistant Secretary for Preparedness
   and Response, Department of Health and Human Services,
   Washington, DC
CHERYL PETERSON, American Nurses Association, Silver Spring,
   MD
SALLY PHILLIPS, Agency for Healthcare Research and Quality,
   Rockville, MD
STEVEN PHILLIPS, National Library of Medicine, Bethesda, MD
EDITH ROSATO, National Association of Chain Drug Stores
   Foundation, Alexandria, VA (since July 2009)
PHILLIP SCHNEIDER, National Association of Chain Drug Stores
   Foundation, Alexandria, VA (until July 2009)
ROSLYNE SCHULMAN, American Hospital Association,
   Washington, DC
DANIEL SOSIN, Centers for Disease Control and Prevention, Atlanta,
   GA
SHARON STANLEY, American Red Cross, Washington, DC
ERIC TONER, University of Pittsburgh Medical Center, Pittsburgh, PA
REED TUCKSON, UnitedHealth Group, Minneapolis, MN
MARGARET VANAMRINGE, The Joint Commission, Washington,
   DC


*IOM Staff*

BRUCE ALTEVOGT, Project Director
CLARE STROUD, Program Officer
ANDREW POPE, Director, Board on Health Sciences Policy
MARNINA KAMMERSELL, Research Associate
ALEX REPACE, Senior Program Assistant

# Reviewers

This report has been reviewed in draft form by individuals chosen for their diverse perspectives and technical expertise, in accordance with procedures approved by the National Research Council's Report Review Committee. The purpose of this independent review is to provide candid and critical comments that will assist the institution in making its published report as sound as possible and to ensure that the report meets institutional standards for objectivity, evidence, and responsiveness to the study charge. The review comments and draft manuscript remain confidential to protect the integrity of the process. We wish to thank the following individuals for their review of this report:

**Roy Alson,** Forsyth County EMS, NC
**Nancy J. Auer,** Swedish Medical Center, WA
**Julie Casani,** North Carolina Division of Public Health
**Linda Degutis,** Yale Center for Public Health Preparedness
**Robert Hood,** Florida Department of Health, Tallahassee

Although the reviewers listed above have provided many constructive comments and suggestions, they did not see the final draft of the report before its release. The review of this report was overseen by **Dr. Kristine M. Gebbie,** School of Nursing, Hunter College City University of New York. Appointed by the Institute of Medicine, she was responsible for making certain that an independent examination of this report was carried out in accordance with institutional procedures and that all review comments were carefully considered. Responsibility for the final content of this report rests entirely with the authoring committee and the institution.

# Contents

INTRODUCTION 1

FORUM AND WORKSHOP OBJECTIVES 2

RELATED IOM WORK ON CRISIS STANDARDS OF CARE 4
Definition of "Crisis Standards of Care," 5
Other Related Work, 5

CRISIS STANDARDS OF CARE PROTOCOLS 6
Developing Crisis Standards of Care Protocols, 8
Who Makes the Plan?, 9

CONTINUUM OF SURGE CAPACITY AND STANDARDS
OF CARE 11
Conventional, Contingency, and Crisis Standards of Care, 12
Stages of Care in the North Dakota Plan, 14

CLINICAL OPERATIONS 15
Indicators, 16
Triggers, 16
Triage, 17
Alternate Care Facilities, 21
Broadening the Scope: Emergency Medical Services, Community
    Health, and Other Components of the Health System, 23
Resource Availability and Distribution, 26
Pediatrics and Other At-Risk Populations, 27
Palliative Care, 28
Mental Health Care, 30
Training, 31

**PROVIDER INVOLVEMENT AND ENGAGEMENT**                    **32**
Engaging Frontline Providers, 32
Hospital Officials, 35

**PUBLIC ENGAGEMENT AND EDUCATION**                        **36**
Changing the Culture of Preparedness, 37
Elected Officials and the Media, 38

**DEVELOPING INTRASTATE AND INTERSTATE
COOPERATION AND CONSISTENCY**                              **39**
FEMA Regions, 41
The All Hazards Consortium, 42
The Interstate Disaster Medical Cooperative, 43
Village-to-Village Communication, 43
Communications and Consistency, 44

**THE ROLE OF THE FEDERAL GOVERNMENT AND
NATIONAL LEADERSHIP**                                      **46**
The Veterans Health Administration, 48
The Department of Defense, 49

**ETHICAL CONSIDERATIONS**                                 **51**

**LEGAL ISSUES FOR CRISIS STANDARDS OF CARE**             **53**
Legal Liability, 53
Credentialing and Scope of Practice, 57
EMTALA and HIPAA, 58
Legal Triage, 60
Education and Training, 61

**CONCLUSION**                                             **61**

**APPENDIXES**

**A**  References                                          65
**B**  Summary of *Guidance for Establishing Crisis Standards
       of Care for Use in Disaster Situations: A Letter Report*   69
**C**  Workshop Agendas                                    95
**D**  Participant Feedback Survey Responses               105
**E**  Biographical Sketches of Workshop Planning Committee
       Members, Invited Speakers, and Panelists           125

# Introduction[1]

The United States faces the real possibility of a catastrophic public health event that involves tens of thousands or hundreds of thousands of victims. Public health emergencies—such as the 2009 H1N1 pandemic, an intentional anthrax release, infectious disease threats such as severe acute respiratory syndrome (SARS), fires, floods, earthquakes, and hurricanes—highlight the ever-changing threats posed by acts of terrorism and other public health emergencies, while also underscoring the pressing reality of these events. A tremendous effort has been made over the past decade to prepare for public health emergencies. Many states and healthcare organizations have developed preparedness plans that include enhancing surge capacity to increase and maximize available resources and to manage demand for healthcare services in response to a mass casualty event.

During a wide-reaching catastrophic public health emergency or disaster, however, these surge capacity plans may not be sufficient to enable healthcare providers to continue to adhere to normal treatment procedures and follow usual standards of care. This is a particular concern for emergencies that may severely strain resources across a large geographic area, such as a pandemic influenza or the detonation of a nuclear device. Healthcare organizations and providers may face overwhelming demand for services, severe scarcity of material resources, insufficient numbers of qualified providers, and too little patient care space. Under these circumstances, it may be impossible to provide care according to the standards of care used in non-disaster situations, and, under the most extreme

---

[1]The planning committee's role was limited to planning the series of regional workshops, and the workshop summary has been prepared by the workshop rapporteurs as a factual summary of what occurred at the regional workshops.

*1*

circumstances, it may not even be possible to provide basic life-sustaining interventions to all patients who need them.

In recent years, a number of federal, state, and local efforts have taken place to develop crisis standards of care protocols and policies for use in conditions of overwhelming resource scarcity. Those involved in these efforts have begun to carefully consider these difficult issues and to develop plans that are ethical, consistent with the community's values, and implementable during a crisis. These planning efforts are essential because, absent careful planning, there is enormous potential for confusion, chaos, and flawed decision making in a catastrophic public health emergency or disaster.

However, although these efforts have accomplished a tremendous amount in just a few years, a great deal remains to be done in even the most advanced plan. Furthermore, the efforts have mainly been taking place independently, leading to a lack of consistency across neighboring jurisdictions and unnecessary duplication of effort. Lastly, many states have not yet substantially begun to develop policies and protocols for crisis standards of care during a mass casualty event.

These issues prompted the Institute of Medicine's (IOM's) Forum on Medical and Public Health Preparedness for Catastrophic Events (Preparedness Forum) to organize a series of regional workshops on this topic. These workshops were held in Irvine, CA; Orlando, FL; New York, NY; and Chicago, IL, between March and May of 2009.

## FORUM AND WORKSHOP OBJECTIVES

The IOM's Preparedness Forum was established to foster dialogue among a broad range of stakeholders—practitioners, policy makers, community members, academics, and others—and to provide ongoing opportunities to confront issues of mutual interest and concern. The Forum provides a neutral venue for broad-ranging policy discussions that can aid in coordination and cooperation between public and private stakeholders in developing and enhancing the nation's medical and public health preparedness. Sponsoring members include federal agencies, state and local associations, health professional associations, and private-sector business associations.

The goals of the workshops on Crisis Standards of Care were to learn from the work already being done to develop state, regional, and local crisis standards of care policies and protocols; to identify areas that require further development, research, and consideration; and to facilitate communication and collaboration among neighboring jurisdictions.

Organized by an independent planning committee, the workshops brought together a wide range of key stakeholders, including policy makers from state and local public health departments; local and regional public health leaders; local and state government representatives; healthcare providers, including representatives of relevant medical disciplines, nursing, pediatrics, emergency medical services (EMS), palliative care, mental health, hospice, and home health; and healthcare and hospital administrators. See Appendix C for workshop agendas and Appendix E for biographical sketches of planning committee members, invited speakers, and panelists. This report is a summary of the presentations and discussions that took place during the workshop. Any opinions, conclusions, or recommendations discussed in this workshop summary are solely those of the individual participants at the workshop and are not necessarily adopted, endorsed, or verified by the Forum or the National Academies.

Workshop speakers and attendees discussed the roles and responsibilities of each stakeholder community in establishing state, regional, and local crisis standards of care protocols. In addition, they were asked to discuss what resources, guidance, and expertise had been established regarding crisis standards of care, including the legal and ethical guidance used to frame those discussions in different localities across the country. Finally, meeting participants were asked to help identify and discuss what resources they needed from federal, state, and regional authorities in order to advance and accelerate the establishment of coordinated and consistent crisis standards of care protocols.

This workshop summary aims to highlight the extensive work that has already been done on this topic across the nation and to raise awareness of current barriers and promising directions for future work. In particular, this document will draw attention to existing federal, state, and local policies and protocols for crisis standards of care; discuss current barriers to increased provider and community engagement; relay examples of existing interstate collaborations; and present workshop participants' ideas, comments, concerns, and potential solutions to some of the most difficult challenges.

## RELATED IOM WORK ON CRISIS STANDARDS OF CARE

This workshop series served as background for a subsequent Institute of Medicine letter report entitled *Guidance for Establishing Crisis Standards of Care for Use in Disaster Situations* (IOM, 2009). This letter report was requested by the Office of the Assistant Secretary for Preparedness and Response (ASPR), Department of Health and Human Services (HHS). The workshop series was organized prior to the onset of the letter report and was not technically part of those efforts. However, the committee that authored the letter report was aware of the information discussed at the regional workshops and this information was subsequently used as one of the key background sources for the committee's work. Consequently, the letter report helped to inform and advance many of the issues that were identified by participants at the workshops.

Unlike this workshop summary, the letter report offers a series of consensus committee recommendations. The report concludes that "[i]n an important ethical sense, entering a crisis standards of care mode is not optional—it is a forced choice, based on the emerging situation. Under such circumstances, failing to make substantive adjustments to care operations—i.e., not to adopt crisis standards of care—is very likely to result in greater death, injury, or illness." The committee also concluded that there is an urgent and clear need for a single national guidance for states with crisis standards of care that can be generalized to all crisis events and is not specific to a certain event. However, the committee recognized that within such a single general framework, individual disaster scenarios may require specific considerations, such as differences between no-notice events and slow-onset events, while the key elements and components remain the same.

The report articulates current concepts and guidance that can assist state and local public health officials, healthcare facilities, and professionals in the development of systematic and comprehensive policies and protocols for crisis standards of care in disasters in which resources are scarce. The committee also identified a series of five key elements and associated components that should be included in all crisis standards of care protocols. Finally, in an extensive "operations" section, the report provides guidance to clinicians, healthcare institutions, and state and local public health officials on how those crisis standards of care should be implemented in a disaster situation. A summary of the committee's recommendations, findings, and practical guidance is included in Appendix

B. The complete letter report is available at http://www.iom.edu/disasterstandards.

## Definition of "Crisis Standards of Care"

For purposes of developing recommendations for situations in which healthcare resources are overwhelmed, in the letter report the IOM committee defined the level of health and medical care capable of being delivered during a catastrophic event as "crisis standards of care":

> "Crisis standards of care" is defined as a substantial change in usual healthcare operations and the level of care it is possible to deliver, which is made necessary by a pervasive (e.g., pandemic influenza) or catastrophic (e.g., earthquake, hurricane) disaster. This change in the level of care delivered is justified by specific circumstances and is formally declared by a state government, in recognition that crisis operations will be in effect for a sustained period. The formal declaration that crisis standards of care are in operation enables specific legal/regulatory powers and protections for healthcare providers in the necessary tasks of allocating and using scarce medical resources and implementing alternate care facility operations.

This definition was developed by the committee that authored the letter report after the workshops took place, and no formal definition was used for the purposes of the workshop. In addition, for consistency this workshop summary uses the term "crisis standards of care" even though this term was only adopted by the IOM after the workshops took place. The remainder of this document outlines the discussions and presentations that took place during the workshops.

## Other Related Work

The IOM letter report and these regional workshops built on a series of previous efforts, many of which were mentioned during the workshops. Workshop attendees praised the work of the Agency for Healthcare Research and Quality (AHRQ) and the Office of the Assistant Secretary for Preparedness and Response for driving the discussion forward. The two agencies came together in 2004 to jumpstart the discussion by convening a panel with experts in the fields of bioethics, emergency medicine, emergency management, health administration, health law and policy, and public health. The result of that meeting was a critical document, *Altered Standards of Care in a Mass Casualty Event*, which served as a foundational document for communities approaching the issues of critical care (AHRQ, 2005).

Producing the document, however, was not easy. "When we first starting working on this subject in 2004, [hospital leaders] wouldn't even agree to sit with us," said Sally Phillips, director of public health emergency preparedness for AHRQ. "Their risk managers wouldn't allow them to come."

A subsequent report, published in 2007 and entitled *Mass Medical Care with Scarce Resources: A Community Planning Guide*, further advanced the field by providing an initial framework for developing policies and protocols for crisis standards of care (Phillips and Knebel, 2007).

Professional societies and academia also have made several recent efforts. Many workshop participants were involved with or highlighted the work undertaken through the American College of Chest Physicians, which resulted in a supplemental issue on the management of mass critical care in the journal *Chest*. This group brought together a multidisciplinary group of experts to provide an in-depth look at current U.S. and Canadian baseline critical care preparedness and response capabilities and limitations, and developed a framework for the development of mass critical care plans. Of particular interest to the workshop participants was the work on allocation of scarce critical care resources (Devereaux et al., 2008). The American Nurses Association (ANA) has also addressed this topic (ANA, 2008; Gebbie et al., 2009).

## CRISIS STANDARDS OF CARE PROTOCOLS

In the past few years, several states have developed policies and protocols for allocation of scarce resources and crisis standards of care. However, these efforts have largely been taking place independently. In fact, many workshop participants expressed surprise at learning how much work had already been done on this topic in states across the nation.

Many panelists and other participants at the workshops were integrally involved in developing those policies and protocols and shared their documents and experiences at the workshops. Among the states that have publicly available protocols are California, Colorado, Massachusetts, Minnesota, New York, Utah, Virginia, and Washington (California Department of Public Health, 2008; Colorado Department of Public Health and Environment, 2009; Levin et al., 2009; Minnesota Department of Health, 2008; Powell et al., 2008; The Commonwealth of Massachusetts Department of Public Health, 2007; The Utah Hospitals and Health Systems Association, 2009; Virginia Department of Health, 2008; Washington State Department of Health's Altered Standards of Care Workgroup, 2008). In Canada, the province of Ontario has also developed crisis standards of care protocols, including particular considerations for patients with cancer or chronic renal disease/acute renal injury, and for blood services and long-term care (Ontario Ministry of Health and Long-term Care, 2008). At the federal level, the Veterans Health Administration (VHA) has developed a protocol for allocation of scarce life-saving resources in VHA during an influenza pandemic (VHA, 2008a, 2009a).

Despite the ongoing work in pockets around the country, it was also clear that most state and local governments and healthcare facilities were in very early stages of developing such policies and protocols or had yet to begin. Among participants who completed the feedback survey after the workshops, just less than half responded that the organization they represented had developed or begun to develop crisis standards of care policies (see Appendix D for the complete set of responses).

At the meeting in Orlando, Kenn Beeman, a senior physician in the Office of Emergency Planning and Response for the Mississippi State Department of Health, discussed significant barriers in his state that have, to date, prohibited the development of crisis standards of care protocols and the engagement of providers in this issue. Among them, "The vast number of Medicare, no-care, no-pay patients [in Mississippi, Arkansas, and West Virginia] places a burden on us from the standpoint of reimbursement," he said. "Philosophically, [many providers] believe that they are already practicing potentially in somewhat of an altered standard of care."

## Developing Crisis Standards of Care Protocols

Many participants at the workshops described efforts under way in their states to begin the discussion about crisis standards of care. In many cases this involved convening a committee or panel of experts to begin to lay the groundwork. For example, in Louisiana the Department of Health and Hospitals organized a Pandemic Influenza Clinical Forum, which was designed to engage a wide variety of healthcare participants to provide guidance to the state as it develops policy and procedural guidelines for crisis standards of care (Box 1). The goal of the group is to use the clinical expertise and knowledge of its members to help develop decision-making steps or matrixes for the ethical distribution of scarce medical resources.

Drawing on the experiences of states already significantly advanced in the process of developing crisis standards of care protocols, the 2009 IOM letter report laid out a five-step process that states could follow to develop such protocols (Appendix B; IOM, 2009). This process, together with the adoption of key elements and components that the committee identified, offers an opportunity to develop a consistent national framework for crisis standards of care.

"The challenge is not to wait for every community in the country to have a disaster befall [its] own citizens, but to figure out how can we proactively move this conversation forward," said Edward Gabriel, the director of global crisis management and business continuity at The Walt Disney Corporation.

---

**BOX 1**
**Louisiana Pandemic Influenza Clinical Forum Priorities**

- Researching existing data/resources
- Planning/collaborating with other states
- Identifying key partners/organizations
- Identifying standards to be addressed
- Identifying the scope of clinical practice
- Developing "triggers" to activate
- Developing an algorithm for allocation of limited resources
- Funding to develop protocols
- Guidance and support from federal authorities

Several workshop participants emphasized that careful advance planning to avoid or mitigate the effects of scarce resources, along with other aspects of effective surge capacity planning, would in fact decrease or delay the need to implement crisis standards of care.

## Who Makes the Plan?

One of the topics discussed in detail at each regional meeting was who should be brought to the table to ensure that the protocols developed are fair and equitable. One of the first steps toward building consensus on fair and ethical crisis standards of care is to bring in all of the parties who have a stake in the discussion. It is not enough, clearly, for a single hospital to have an established plan for how it will handle resource shortages. Those plans must be shared and coordinated across regional lines to prevent the kind of "hospital shopping" that could cause chaos and further overwhelm the system. Participants discussed the importance of bringing political and community leaders and members of the media into the fold and encouraging them to reach out to their communities to educate, inform, and, if necessary, guide appropriate behavior. Many participants also stressed that the community must be engaged, emergency medical experts consulted, and external providers such as pharmacists and insurance providers enlisted in the cause.

However, one lesson that emerged from the workshops is that the list of groups that should be involved and engaged in the planning process is much bigger even than this (Box 2). Deborah Levy, chief of health preparedness for the Centers for Disease Control and Prevention (CDC), described a program in which the CDC works with a community to develop a model for healthcare delivery during a public health crisis. Communities are selected based on a set of criteria, one of which is the level of collaboration between public health and the various components of the healthcare sector. "We want 911 and other call centers, emergency medical services, emergency departments, hospital administrators, public health, primary care providers, urgent care and other outpatient clinics, long-term care and skilled nursing facilities, hospice and palliative care, home health organizations, pharmacists, emergency management, local government such as mayors, and VA [Veterans Administration] and DoD [Department of Defense] facilities if they happen to be in your community," said Levy. "We usually require at least three representatives from each of those sectors to be at the table and over a 2½-day time period . . . to think through how they'd deliver care."

Others added further to that list, including groups traditionally considered completely outside the healthcare field, such as funeral directors and morticians.

The reason for including all these different participants in planning goes deeper than the simple practicality of integrating care.

"If you're doing this kind of emergency planning . . . every institution needs to be represented," said Gabriel of The Walt Disney Corporation. "Otherwise they will sit back after you are done and say that they had no involvement." Gabriel noted that the lack of participation paves the way for outsiders to criticize the difficult decisions when the time comes. That makes it particularly critical to capture the buy-in of both hospital leadership and politicians.

---

**BOX 2**
**Who Should Participate in Planning**
**for Crisis Standards of Care? A Partial List**

- Physicians
- Physician assistants
- Nurses
- Nurse practitioners
- EMTs/paramedics and dispatchers
- Pharmacists
- Hospital administrators
- State and local public health officials
- Emergency management
- Fire departments
- Police departments
- Ethicists
- Lawyers
- Morticians
- Funeral directors
- Citizens
- Elected officials
- Media
- Bloggers
- Teachers

- Large local employers
- Faith-based organizations
- Civic organizations
- Academia
- Charities and nonprofits
- Government
- Insurance companies
- Reinsurance companies
- Hospitals and hospital associations
- Nursing facilities
- Health system alliances
- Veterans Affairs hospitals
- Department of Defense facilities
- Community health centers
- Urgent care facilities
- Hospice and palliative care facilities
- Long-term care facilities
- Home health organizations
- Dialysis centers
- Hospital licensing agencies
- Regulatory agencies

In order to facilitate this broad involvement in Utah, the Governor's Public Health Emergency Preparedness Advisory Council convenes partners from government, health care, and the private sector in the governor's executive boardroom. Members of the council are appointed by the governor. "People have a hard time saying they won't come when they know they're in his own executive boardroom, and that makes it very effective for us," said Paul Patrick, director of the Bureau of EMS and Preparedness in the Utah Department of Health.

Even while stressing the importance of engaging a wide range of stakeholders, several workshop participants also emphasized the importance of leadership and the use of effective procedures to ensure that the planning process does not become unwieldy. The 2009 IOM letter report outlines a five-step process that state public health authorities can use to develop crisis standards of care protocols (IOM, 2009). The process uses a series of working groups and committees to outline ethical considerations, review legal authority, and draft guidance. This is followed by a broad public stakeholder engagement process, after which the ethical elements and crisis standards of care can be finalized, incorporating changes raised during the engagement process, as appropriate. The final step of the process is the establishment of a Medical Disaster Advisory Committee that will provide ongoing advice to the state authority regarding changes to the situation and potential corresponding changes in the implementation of crisis standards of care. In this way, the process incorporates both broad stakeholder and public engagement as well as smaller groups that can function effectively to draft, refine, and provide real-time advice about implementation.

## CONTINUUM OF SURGE CAPACITY AND STANDARDS OF CARE

Many workshop participants stressed that making changes to usual standards of care is not an all-or-none situation. The changes required depend on the nature and extent of the disaster, the existing capabilities of the community, and the particular resources that become scarce, among many other variables. Several participants emphasized that the response to the disaster should be proportional, and changes to standards of care should be the minimum necessary given the circumstances.

Efforts to define a common taxonomy and framework for discussion are a first step to ensuring a proportional response, to developing protocols that are sufficiently detailed so as to be implementable, and to begin the discussion of exactly when healthcare providers and facilities should implement crisis standards of care.

## Conventional, Contingency, and Crisis Standards of Care

John Hick, associate medical director for EMS and medical director of emergency preparedness at Hennepin County Medical Center, MN, presented a framework from an article published in the June 2009 issue of the *Journal of Disaster Medicine and Public Health Preparedness* (Hick et al., 2009). Hick and his coauthors described three categories of surge capacity: conventional capacity, contingency capacity, and crisis capacity (Box 3). The description resonated strongly with workshop participants and came to define the discussions of care at each of the workshops. The recent IOM committee on crisis standards of care also adopted this terminology and framework (IOM, 2009).

"Conventional capacity is really about providing patient care without any change in daily practice," said Hick. Most hospitals and other healthcare resources can face small surges in demand, but still operate within the conventional framework. They may cancel elective surgeries, or accelerate the discharge of healthy patients, but they will still perform invasive procedures in standard operating rooms, follow standard protocols, and generally operate in a business-as-usual mindset. Staff may be asked to pitch in and support different areas of the hospital—a trauma surgeon may be pulled into the emergency room—but staff will not be operating outside of their bounds of expertise.

"As you move into contingency modes of reaction, you're starting to . . . change practice a little, but it still really doesn't have any significant impact on the care delivered or on the outcomes achieved," said Hick.

Contingency care might mean using rooms of the hospital for different kinds of clinical care than usual, such as using post-anesthesia care rooms or procedure areas for care that would usually be delivered in an intensive care unit (ICU). Practitioners may start conserving supplies by, for example, not providing precautionary oxygen to patients who under normal circumstances would receive it, but who can survive and recover without it.

"As we move into the crisis level, we're really starting to make some pretty substantial changes to the way we provide care, and there are some implications for patient outcomes," said Hick. "We're trying to do the best we can with the resources available."

In crisis situations, staff may be asked to practice outside of the scope of their usual expertise. Supplies may have to be reused and recycled. In some circumstances, resources may become completely exhausted. Family members may be asked to provide basic patient hygiene and other aspects of care that do not require medical expertise.

"Crisis capacity is really defined as adapting spaces, staff, and resources so that . . . you're doing the best you can with what you have," said Dan Hanfling, special advisor to the Inova Health System in Falls Church, VA, on matters related to emergency preparedness and disaster response. "You're providing the best possible care under the circumstances."

As Hick noted, the goal is always to avoid entering contingency or crisis care. However, if that becomes unavoidable and a facility is operating under contingency or crisis care, the goal is "to get back to a conventional footing." Hick discussed strategies of preparation, substitution, adaptation, conservation, reuse, and finally, reallocation. Strategies that have a lesser impact on clinical care, such as substitution, should be used first, and strategies such as reallocation should be used only when other strategies have not been sufficient to address the resource shortage. He

---

**BOX 3**
**Continuum of Conventional, Contingency, and Crisis Capacity**

**Conventional capacity:** The spaces, staff, and supplies used are consistent with daily practices within the institution. These spaces and practices are used during a major mass casualty incident that triggers activation of the facility emergency operations plan.

**Contingency capacity:** The spaces, staff, and supplies used are not consistent with daily practices, but maintain or have minimal impact on usual patient care practices. These spaces or practices may be used temporarily during a major mass casualty incident or on a more sustained basis during a disaster (when the demands of the incident exceed community resources).

**Crisis capacity:** Adaptive spaces, staff, and supplies are not consistent with usual standards of care, but provide sufficiency of care in the setting of a catastrophic disaster (i.e., provide the best possible care to patients given the circumstances and resources available) (Hick et al., 2009).

---

highlighted a set of informational cards for healthcare providers and institutions that he and others developed in Minnesota that lays out patient care strategies for scarce resource situations (Minnesota Department of Health, 2008). The card set lists appropriate substitution, adaptation, conservation, reuse, and reallocation strategies for oxygen, medication administration, hemodynamic support and IV fluids, mechanical ventilation, nutrition, and staffing.

## Stages of Care in the North Dakota Plan

Officials in the state of North Dakota have also outlined incremental changes to standards of care. During the Chicago workshop, Tim Wiedrich, chief of emergency preparedness and response for the North Dakota Department of Health, presented their work on outlining levels of care (Box 4).

Stage 1 involves a small shift in patient care that may inconvenience some patients, but will not have a measurable impact on patient care. It is akin to the "conventional" care category outlined by Hick.

As an event escalates, North Dakota moves into Stage II, taking steps that limit the quality of care and may impact patient outcomes. Doctors and nurses are asked to operate slightly outside their normal bounds of expertise, retired caregivers are called back onto the job, and changes are made in standard operating procedures such as charting and checking vital signs.

Stage III is akin to the crisis care scenario outlined by Hick and others. In a Stage III emergency, the North Dakota system operates under a "best efforts" basis that attempts to stretch the medical response to serve as many patients as possible. At Stage III, the impact on care is severe. A decision such as "no CPR" has real consequences, but in this scenario is deemed necessary to ensure the best possible care is delivered to the maximum number of people.

---

**BOX 4**
**Stages of Care in North Dakota's Plan**

**STAGE 1: SMALL OUTCOME IMPACT**

- Tighter admission criteria
- Early discharge
- Eliminate comfort-care nursing
- Increase shift length
- Small increases in patient-to-provider ratio

- Eliminate dietary preference
- Limited post-mortem care
- Hospital access restriction
- Cohorting

**STAGE II: MODERATE OUTCOME IMPACT**

- Acute care remains at nursing homes
- Limitations in services, diagnostics
- Limited expansion of privileges
- Moderate increase in patient-to-provider ratio
- Provider recruitment (e.g., retired)

- Increased care by family members
- Decreased frequency of vital signs
- Changes in palliative care
- Changes in charting

**STAGE III: SEVERE OUTCOME IMPACT**

- Marked expansion in privileges
- Large increase in patient-to-provider ratio
- Use of volunteers for some patient care
- Family administration of medications
- Palliative threshold increase (low survival conditions)

- No cardiopulmonary resuscitation
- Clinical judgment replaces diagnostics
- Changes in informed consent requirements
- Minimal charting

---

# CLINICAL OPERATIONS

The decision to implement crisis standards of care is a significant event—it changes how hospitals and caregivers operate, it changes the legal environment, and it changes citizen expectations. A significant portion of the workshops was devoted to how and when that decision would be made, and how hospitals should implement crisis standards of care.

## Indicators

Implementation of crisis standards of care first requires recognition of an actual or impending resource shortfall. Workshop participants noted that many different resources may become scarce at different times, depending on the nature of the disaster and the characteristics of the community and the healthcare facility. The 2009 IOM report listed the following resources as likely to be scarce in a crisis care environment and possibly justifying specific planning and tracking:

- Ventilators and components
- Oxygen and oxygen delivery devices
- Vascular access devices
- Intensive care unit beds
- Healthcare providers, particularly critical care, burn, and surgical/anesthesia staff (nurses and physicians) and respiratory therapists
- Hospitals (due to infrastructure damage or compromise)
- Specialty medications or IV fluids (sedatives/analgesics, specific antibiotics, antivirals, etc.)
- Vasopressors/inotropes
- Medical transportation

Workshop participants emphasized that it was important that healthcare facilities be aware of impending shortages so they could take steps to avoid having to implement crisis standards of care. Participants also noted the importance of having situational awareness of the system because the entire network of indicators will provide the most accurate sense of the level of stress on the system. For example, a shortage of ventilators will be compensated by the use of other ventilator processes, in turn making those supplies scarce for their originally specified use. In this way, a small number of significantly scarce resources can cause strain throughout the entire system.

## Triggers

To achieve integrated, consistent, and fair care, every participant in the system must be operating with the same understanding of where things stand on the conventional/contingency/crisis scale. In fact, many workshop members indicated the need for multiple triggers operating at different levels and with different time frames.

Speaking of his own experience in New York, David Hoffman from Wyckoff Heights Medical Center said his group identified the need for multiple triggers. "There needs to be a trigger based on the declaration of disaster from government officials if there is a statewide or regional event," Hoffman suggested. "There needs to be a trigger at an institutional level so that there is the means of communicating to the staff that . . . a new set of rules applied. . . . And what we've learned from the situation in Katrina . . . is that there needs to be a factual trigger that can be applied retroactively" to provide legal protection for caregivers.

Some participants believed those triggers should be driven on the scene by frontline staff. "I think those kinds of triggers need to be defined by the people who are on the front lines and will be forced to make those decisions," said HHS's Rear Admiral Ann Knebel. "We need to support them and make sure that there is, as much as possible, consistency in terms of the principles that drive what those triggers are." Knebel said that the trigger point comes when available resources are no longer adequate to support patient demand.

Different states have taken different approaches to determining who should make the decision, some empowering governors and others looking to public health officials to help define the triggers and determine the mechanism for transitioning from normal to crisis standards of care. However, as the 2009 IOM report concluded, working through a framework that begins at the institutional and local levels, the authority to institute crisis standards of care lies with the state. In most states, the state department of health holds this responsibility. Some states have well-defined processes for establishing their protocols, but many others are still in development.

## Triage

Once a determination has been made that conventional care standards no longer apply, workshop participants commented, the rapid implementation of an effective triage program should be one of the first goals of any healthcare program. A triage program aims to rapidly screen, evaluate, and sort patients based on their medical status and likely outcome.

Ken Berkowitz from the Veterans Administration National Center for Ethics explained a working model of the VHA Hospitals' operating protocol during pandemic influenza: "Our tertiary triage protocol is the process of sorting acute care hospital patients into three treatment groups. Initial decisions are based on survivability, and that's justified by the goal of making optimum use of resources and meeting the goal of overall population health. Second-order decisions for equally prioritized patients are based on a first-come, first-served basis, or if that's not possible, on a lottery basis. That is justified by the principle of fairness."

As many participants noted, the triage process outlined in the American College of Chest Physicians work on mass critical care has formed the basis for the protocols developed by the VHA and many of the states (Colorado Department of Public Health and Environment, 2009; Devereaux et al., 2008; IOM, 2009; Minnesota Department of Health, 2008; The Utah Hospitals and Health Systems Association, 2009; VHA, 2008a, 2009a). This triage process includes the use of the Sequential Organ Failure Assessment (SOFA) score for determining triage priorities. The system uses a variety of measures linked to six major organ systems— (1) cardiovascular, (2) coagulation, (3) hepatic, (4) neurological, (5) renal, and (6) respiratory—and is already in use in multiple hospitals. The SOFA scores help triage teams rapidly determine how sick people are, and are relatively easy for hospitals to execute and record. The IOM report's basic triage process is outlined in Figure 1 and exclusion criteria are described in Box 5.

Under this triage process, both patients who score too high and too low on the SOFA assessment are not given critical care resources during an emergency: patients who score too high because they will not likely benefit from medical care, and patients who score too low because they will likely survive without substantial care.

Many workshop participants also emphasized that the use of SOFA scores is far from the perfect solution. "From a pragmatic standpoint, on an individual–patient level, to say that this person is getting resources and this person is not based on a one-point difference on a SOFA score . . . that's a huge issue and something we think about very carefully," said Hennepin County Medical Center's Hick.

Moreover, SOFA scores may not apply to some of the most vulnerable patient groups. Stephen Cantrill, an emergency physician in Colorado, noted that SOFA hasn't been studied in pediatrics, and is not designed as a predictive tool. Many workshop participants noted that the lack of research on SOFA scores and other potential decision tools in pediatric populations is a significant gap and emphasized that much more research should be done in this area so that it can better inform important policy decisions.

Hick said his hospital had an appeals process whereby a patient's physician could appeal back to the triage team for a rescoring if a patient's condition changed.

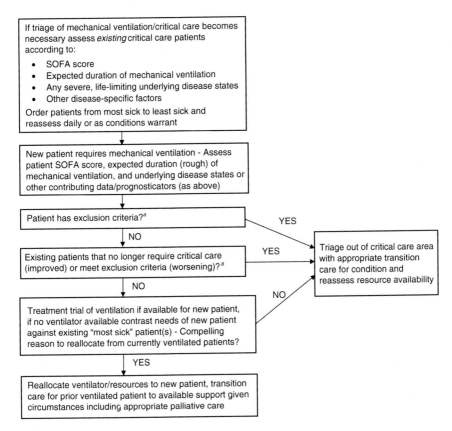

**FIGURE 1** Triage algorithm process.
[a]Example exclusion criteria include severe, irreversible organ failure (congestive heart failure, liver failure, etc.), severe neurologic compromise, extremely high or not improving sequential organ failure assessment (SOFA) scores, etc.
SOURCE: IOM (2009) (adapted from Devereaux et al., 2008).

---

**BOX 5**
**Exclusion Criteria Prompting Possible Reallocation of**
**Life-Saving Interventions**

**Sequential Organ Failure Assessment (SOFA) score criteria:**
patients excluded from critical care if risk of hospital mortality > 80%
A. SOFA > 15
B. SOFA > 5 for >5 d, and with flat or rising trend
C. > 6 organ failures

**Severe, chronic disease with a short life expectancy**
A.  Severe trauma
B.  Severe burns on patient with any two of the following:
    i.  Age > 60 yr
    ii.  > 40% of total body surface area affected
    iii.  Inhalational injury
C.  Cardiac arrest
    i.  Unwitnessed cardiac arrest
    ii.  Witnessed cardiac arrest, not responsive to electrical therapy (defibrillation or pacing)
    iii.  Recurrent cardiac arrest
D.  Severe baseline cognitive impairment
E.  Advanced untreatable neuromuscular disease
F.  Metastatic malignant disease
G.  Advanced and irreversible neurologic event or condition
H.  End-stage organ failure (for details, see Devereaux et al., 2008)
I.  Age > 85 yr (see Lieberman et al., 2009)
J.  Elective palliative surgery

SOURCE: IOM (2009) (adapted from Devereaux et al., 2008).

---

*Triage Across the Health System*

Hospital-level triage, however, is really only one piece of the puzzle. "I would encourage us to be very inclusive in our language," advised Cheryl Peterson, director of nursing practice and policy at the ANA, speaking at the Orlando workshop. "It is not only physicians who do triage. It is your mental health provider. It is your registered nurse. It could be your respiratory therapist. There are a whole host of providers out there who are responsible for making some very difficult decisions, and as we think about our planning, every one of these providers has to be engaged in that decision."

Others discussed the need for a focus on triage at all stages of care. In the Colorado protocol, "We tried to address things from the beginning to the end, starting with telephone triage," said Cantrill. "That's trying to get some standard approach to telephone triage because we know that's going to be a hot area of heightened importance during any type of pandemic."

EMS triage is another area that needs to be aggressively studied, but hasn't. "From the EMS level, we have to decide the basic issues of triage," said North Carolina EMS's Roy Alson. "Who's going to get an ambulance? Who gets transported to the non-hospital care facility?"

Training was another important factor emphasized by workshop participants, who cited the practice in some emergency departments to have "Triage Tuesdays," where all patients are run through the triage system to keep the process fresh in the minds of all practitioners involved.

### Alternate Care Facilities

Most surge capacity plans contain some means of providing non-critical care outside of the hospital setting to free up as many hospital beds as possible for more seriously ill patients. This can take the form of either formal, dedicated facilities that are idle most of the time, or of convertible public spaces such as schools, restaurants, houses of worship, or meeting halls. These facilities are important components of a surge plan, but they raise additional questions regarding crisis standards of care because the facilities may have different staffing levels, make greater use of volunteers or providers practicing outside of their duties, and have more limited care capabilities. Although this was not discussed in great detail at the workshops, participants also mentioned a number of additional challenges related to establishing alternate care facilities, including facility licensing and reimbursement.

"We have bought, thanks to a grant, a 250-bed surge-capacity facility. . . . The beds and everything are in trailers and we can move them to a church hall or to a school gym," said John Robinson, discussing Baptist Memorial Hospital in northern Mississippi's approach to prestaged surge capacity.

Others cautioned that, even if adequate additional resources are available, these facilities must be adequately staffed or they will not function. "We've got eight very nice tractor-trailer-mounted disaster hospitals," said North Carolina's Alson. But "nobody is going to be able to staff them [in a true pandemic]. This is not a hurricane where it's going to go for 4 or 5 weeks maybe. This is months and it's going to be in multiple events and you're going to do it with half your staff eventually."

Workshop participants considered staffing these facilities with a combination of full-time health care physicians, retired physicians, nurse practitioners, and other providers. Many noted that providing palliative care in a surge facility was one area where retired healthcare workers could provide excellent support during a crisis.

In North Dakota, alternate care facilities will provide such care and be staffed by volunteer providers, according to a presentation by North Dakota's Wiedrich. He detailed the basic capabilities that alternate care facilities in North Dakota would provide (Box 6).

Rick Hong, medical director for public health preparedness in the Delaware Division of Public Health, discussed the model for alternate care facilities being used in Delaware (Box 7). He detailed how each component of the system would be staffed, and what kinds of treatments would be available in each.

---

**BOX 6**
**North Dakota Alternate Care Facility Capabilities**

- Hydration
- Nutrition
- Hygiene
- No public access
- Volunteer providers

- Nasogastric hydration
- No IV meds
- Limited nasogastric meds
- No oxygen available
- Include palliative and recovery care

---

**BOX 7**
**Modular Medical Expansion: An Example from Delaware**

The surge program in Delaware is based on a concept called "modular medical expansion." When developing the program, all the parties involved agreed that simply sending all the patients to the hospital was untenable, so they set up a triad of facilities to provide approach care.

The first piece of that triad is Neighborhood Emergency Health Centers, or NEHCs. The NEHCs are located in communities and are designed to handle triage and to function as the gateway for patients into the healthcare system.

"We're relying on historical data stating that most of the patients affected in a disaster do not need medical care or do not need critical care, about 50-80 percent," said Rick Hong, medical director for public health preparedness in the Delaware Division of Public Health. "So our concept is if we can identify those patients first and remove them from the healthcare system, then we'll be able to manage the situation."

The NEHC will be able to provide simple care such as distributing vaccines or antiviral medication. It will be staffed by public health nurses, pharmacists, and other healthcare providers who may not usually see patients. These providers currently undergo annual training to prepare to staff these areas.

Patients identified as needing more significant medical care at the NEHCs will be sent to either an Acute Care Center or a hospital.

The Acute Care Centers are out-of-hospital care settings that are capable of providing a limited array of supportive care to patients in need: IV antibiotics, IV pain medication, IV fluids, and nebulizer treatments. The list of available treatments is intentionally kept small so that these Acute Care Centers can be staffed by non-specialists. Hospitals are required to staff these centers by donating care providers.

"The hospitals said, 'There's no way we're going to be able to give you staff,'" said Hong. "Our response was, 'OK, we'll just send the patients to you. How do you like that?' And they [all agreed] to give staff members."

With NEHCs and the Acute Care Centers siphoning off a large portion of the potential patient population, Delaware's hospitals can be reserved to providing crisis care to the truly ill.

To make the system function, Delaware has put in place laws that limit the liability of providers operating in this situation, and that allow healthcare professionals to expand outside their traditional scope of practice, such as allowing pharmacists to administer vaccines to patients or emergency medical technicians to provide pills.

## Broadening the Scope:
## Emergency Medical Services, Community Health, and Other Components of the Health System

One reality driven home by the workshops is that the forces involved in disaster preparedness are almost, by definition, top-heavy. While the regional workshops brought together a wide array of professions—public health officers, physicians, hospital administrators, researchers, nurses, and emergency medical technicians (EMTs), to name but a few—most planning and policy work on crisis standards of care is focused on the hospital or hospital-network level.

The reason is simple: These larger and more sophisticated healthcare networks are often the only ones with the resources to spend on disaster preparedness. Unfortunately, this top-heavy approach runs counter to the actual nature of responses to medical emergencies.

"Most emergency responses are an upside-down pyramid," noted Kathryn Brinsfield, associate chief medical officer at the Department of Homeland Security (DHS). "Critical care patients are a very small piece of that, and the outpatient care, visiting nurses, all the other places" are crucial.

*Emergency Medical Services*

One recurring theme throughout the workshops was the critical role that the emergency medical services play in directing emergency response, and the limited extent to which they have been incorporated into planning for crisis standards of care.

During day-to-day operations, EMS systems have a mandate to transport individual patients to the closest available hospital, while providing stabilizing care along the way. But as Leslee Stein-Spencer, a Registered Nurse and manager at the Chicago Fire Department, told the Chicago workshop, that approach won't work during a mass casualty situation.

In a mass casualty situation, EMTs may be called on to transfer multiple patients at a single time, to provide medicine to limit infection, to triage patients onsite, or to transport only those who meet certain qualifications. EMTs may be asked to operate outside their standard scope of practice, or transport patients to alternate care facilities. But so far, at least in her region, training and preparation have overlooked this critical link (Box 8).

---

**BOX 8**
**Status of Emergency Medical Services Preparedness in Chicago**

| Issue | Status |
|---|---|
| • Using alternative treatment modalities | • Not being addressed in planning |
| • Creating alternative staffing patterns | • Work has started |
| • Expanding scope of practice | • Work has started |
| • Procedures to transport to alternative facilities | • Not being addressed in planning |

Stein-Spencer identified a series of issues that must be addressed in developing the emergency response, including the following:

- Defining credentialing/licensing activities, both local and state
- Determining the trigger for crisis standards and identifying who makes the call: local, regional, state
- Finalizing mutual aid agreements
- Handling the differences between private and public responders
- Ensuring the consistency of care in adjacent communities

Some participants also noted the special challenges that arise in many communities, particularly rural areas, in which EMS units are largely or entirely volunteer.

### Community Health Centers and Other Resources

Like EMS, community health centers and other "boots on the ground" facilities are also often overlooked in the planning process. But the need to coordinate their care with hospital settings to ensure a single, unified approach to standards is critical.

Kevin McCulley, emergency preparedness coordinator at the Association for Utah Community Health, emphasized that these community health centers represent a largely untapped resource for planners, and could be called on in a pinch to provide critical care space on a short-term basis.

### Private Sector

Large corporations and other private entities must also be brought into the discussion as well, participants said, as they can have outsized influence over disseminating information regarding emergency response and standards of care in an emergency setting. One of the four workshops, in fact, was hosted by a private company—the Orlando meeting was hosted at a Disney resort—reflecting an increased recognition by the private sector that managing these kinds of situations is critical to business continuity.

"Many large corporations are willing to engage in preparedness planning," noted Knebel. "It makes good business sense, and they are part of the community."

## Resource Availability and Distribution

Workshop participants said that identifying available resources is an essential part of laying the foundation for a sound approach to standards of care. Does a hospital know how many emergency beds or emergency ventilators are available? If not, that kind of resource survey should be among the first orders of business when creating a surge program.

William Fales, associate professor of emergency medicine at Michigan State University's Kalamazoo Center for Medical Studies, discussed the work of the Great Lakes Healthcare Partnership to identify the resources available for surge care during an emergency situation. They identified and categorized 123 types of resources available in the region, consolidating those resources into a centralized database that could be used in emergencies.

"It's incumbent on every state and community and planning group to know what your resources are so you can figure out how you're going to fill and meet that gap," said Knebel of HHS.

Davis Tornabene of Sarasota Memorial Hospital, FL, described what she learned in the planning process. "When we did our tabletop regarding pan flu some issues came to light . . . we had really no idea of the state supply of available ventilators, antivirals, things like that," she said.

Others wondered how hospitals could learn more about available resources in the Strategic National Stockpile, such as the numbers and types of ventilators available during a crisis. Although that information may be classified, there were calls to have at least some basic information shared so hospitals could do facility planning.

A broader point made about resources was the need to ensure a fair and adequate distribution of resources, based on processes that can be upheld even as situations become turbulent. "You need those triggers to determine when you're going to say [to hospital distributors] that you can't distribute all your N95 respirators to the hospitals that are paying you the most money," said HHS's Knebel. "You have to make sure you distribute them to those people who don't go to those hospitals, the people who live in the inner cities."

It is all too easy to imagine hospitals hoarding supplies, or suppliers demanding ever higher prices for the remaining few doses of a particular drug. In Colorado, one workshop participant offered, draft orders were under consideration that would allow the governor to seize supplies from any location and redistribute them to other locations.

When supplies do run out, a number of participants suggested developing guidelines for how to reuse and recycle spent resources. Studies are needed, they suggested, on how long supplies such as surgical masks can be used before being discarded in suboptimal environments. In an environment focused on doing the greatest good for the greatest number, extracting the maximum value from limited supplies is crucial.

## Pediatrics and Other At-Risk Populations

If crisis standards of care are to be fair, particular attention must be paid to planning for at-risk populations such as children and older adults, workshop participants noted. The challenges of basic triage multiply in these populations for a variety of reasons. There is less available research on which to base decisions, and the care required may be more specialized so even during non-disaster times there are fewer trained healthcare providers and appropriate resources. There is also the potential that a communications problem or a lack of understanding of the special needs of people with disabilities such as sight or hearing impairments could impact the triage process. In some cases, the decisions are simply more emotional.

"Large-scale pediatric casualties could be more than we could bear," warned George Foltin, speaking of his work on emergency planning with the New York City Department of Health, at the meeting in the Bronx. When triaging pediatric patients, "we need to think of this sometimes as if we were wartime England. We need to be brave. We need to make correct choices. We need to protect our way of life and we need to focus on our children." Most hospital settings do not have the specialty equipment or specially trained doctors to provide surge coverage of pediatric patients, Foltin noted. As a result, "The major pediatric center must surge," he said. "We think that critically ill and injured children are better off at a major center that has [the equipment and expertise] to take care of them, even under less than optimal circumstances, rather than going to a hospital that doesn't know how to take care of them."

Children represent 25 percent of the U.S. population, so our failure to plan explicitly for their care represents an acute failure of overall planning.

Children, of course, are not the only ones. In fact, there may be situations where the rest of the population is carrying on as normal even as a special-population care facility is completely overwhelmed. "A perfect example was the [New York City] blackout in 2003," added Judith Ahronheim, a New York geriatrician. "We were thinking about terrorism, but the largest number of admissions to the hospital was vulnerable elderly people whose electrical appliances had failed."

Mental health patients are another vulnerable population that deserves special attention and care. Anticipating and responding to those needs is a critical part of maintaining a fair standard of care. The importance of upholding fairness during the development and implementation of crisis standards of care is discussed in greater detail below in the section on Ethical Considerations.

Finally, Phillips, of AHRQ, highlighted pregnant women as another group of vulnerable patients. "We don't really want pregnant healthy women going into some of the hospitals during pandemic influenza," said Phillips. But how do we encourage woman to deliver at home in contrast to the broader push for hospital births over the past few decades?

## Palliative Care

Ultimately, despite surge capacity, despite stretching resources, and despite best efforts, the implementation of crisis standards of care in a mass casualty event may mean that some patients will not have access to critical care resources.

Workshop participants widely believed that no patient, regardless of the circumstance, should simply be "left to die." Participants stressed that care is never withdrawn. Patients who are not offered access to critical life-sustaining resources should receive the best available palliative care. Participants also discussed regular reevaluation of patients to see if improving conditions have increased their likelihood of responding to more aggressive treatment using available resources.

These situations "contemplate a context where there will be many, many deaths among people who receive critical care resources, and among those who don't, so it puts an enormous emphasis on palliative care," said Tia Powell, director of the Montefiore-Einstein Center for Bioethics in The Bronx, New York.

Despite the obvious need, participants worried that too little had been done to establish protocols and standards for palliative care for those who do not receive life sustaining resources. So much energy is spent worrying about resource allocation for those patients who *do* receive critical care resources that almost none is left over for those who don't. "It's distressing after this many years that there's still a reluctance to talk about palliative care," said Knebel from the HHS. Even in healthcare circles, there's a reluctance to admit that sometimes the best the healthcare system can do is to make a patient more comfortable.

"It's a perfectly acceptable standard of care in the appropriate situation," said Jan Rhyne of the North Carolina Medical Board, who thought it should not even qualify as a crisis standard of care. "It is a very noble type of care, and I think the hospitals are having a tough time getting that message out right now."

Workshop participants highlighted the need for extensive work on how patients should be treated if life-sustaining treatment such as ventilator support is not offered or is discontinued. Similarly, caregivers should be taught how to deal with the stress of these situations, and to handle the very real potential mental health challenges of those involved.

"I find that personally, in the circles I travel in [palliative care] is now the new third rail of disaster medicine," said Inova's Hanfling. "We can talk somewhat comfortably about this shift in standards of care . . . but when we talk about palliative care . . . withdrawing ongoing life support—you know it is really frowned upon and I get a lot of push back."

The decision to reallocate life-sustaining treatment from one patient in favor of another is a very real, on-the-ground issue in a mass casualty situation. "How do you manage that transition?" asks Minnesota's Hick. "You're in the ICU, [the patient is] on the ventilator, and now you extubate the person. . . . Do you keep the patient there? . . . Do you have a palliative care area you move them to? What kind of support do they have? Those are exactly the kinds of issues we need to think through."

The scenario is even more basic than that. "There's virtually no standard protocols for external extubation in the literature now. I mean, there was something in *Chest Soundings* a few years ago, but there's very little for non-pandemic standards of how to do it. So that's just an existing gap, period," noted Berkowitz from the VHA.

These are not easy issues. In the context of a mass casualty event, palliative care may be given to patients who, in normal situations, would receive aggressive interventions and potentially life-sustaining therapies. Exactly how, where, and when to provide this care—and the preparations that must be made to ensure that care is as good as possible—was an area identified as needing significant research.

## Mental Health Care

One area that to date has received little attention is the mental health consequences surrounding some of the hardest decisions contemplated— such as removing ventilator assistance from a patient or ceasing pediatric resuscitations in the field. "One of the things we don't do very well is understand how [practitioners] are likely to respond," said Jack Herrmann, senior advisor for public health preparedness at the National Association of County and City Health Officials. "We plan for how we want them to respond, and less for how they do respond."

The long-term fallout on practitioners and patients will also be great, and multiple participants voiced the need to prepare ahead of time to assist patients and caregivers coping with post-event stress. "When people are going to live in this environment for any period of time, the providers are going to need a lot of support," said Phillips. "They're going to have to live with these decisions. And I think that's something we haven't paid much attention to."

"Grief management's going to be a huge, huge component . . . not just for the individuals who are falling victim to this, but also to the providers who are not able to provide the kind of care and treatment that they feel is important," said David Fleming, professor of Clinical Medicine and the Director of the Center for Health Ethics at the University of Missouri School of Medicine. To meet this need, Missouri is developing just-in-time pandemic grief training for managers and supervisors.

Robert Hood, an ethicist at the Florida Department of Health, noted that Johns Hopkins University has a CDC funding allotment to work on ethical issues and mental health preparedness.

The broader population will also face significant mental health issues. "The community is going to have to deal with families having family members die in their homes [when] normally they would have had a hospice provider maybe coming in and helping them. They may not have that kind of support," noted Phillips. "I think there are a whole lot of implications for the mental health field and mental health providers."

## Training

One challenge that workshop participants consistently noted was the difficulty in effectively training and building relationships across organizational boundaries. Efforts like Levy's community-based CDC workshops help, but the need was identified to develop opportunities that would build ongoing, hands-on, face-to-face relationships among stakeholders before disaster strikes. That means holding joint training exercises and developing personal relationships so that, when disaster does strike, lines of communication will be open.

Inova's Hanfling noted that "planned disasters" can often provide a framework for exactly this kind of discussion. Hanfling noted that the 2009 presidential inauguration provided an opportunity for representatives from Maryland, Virginia, and the District of Columbia to sit together in an emergency operations center ready to manage an emergency response. This enabled them to provide information in real time from their respective jurisdictions, and in turn to communicate information back from the emergency operations center.

Ultimately, no major events occurred during the Inauguration that required a community-wide response. But bringing people together to sit at the same actual table and build relationships was seen as a major and significant step forward. "One of the things that, even for communities that are fairly advanced [in their preparedness planning] . . . is that it is quite interesting when you bring these groups together," said the CDC's Levy. "For one, they usually end up realizing that they don't really know the details of each other's plans, or they're making assumptions that turn out to be incorrect, or someone will have a plan and another group didn't even know they had that plan. Also hospital leaderships, we've found, usually haven't grasped the complexity of the issues that are involved in these types of mass events."

As these diverse groups are brought together, however, there is a need to mediate the situation and foster a fair discussion. These *are* difficult issues, and tensions *can* be high.

"I would encourage everybody to look at having a neutral, outside moderator when you bring your core group together," said Roy Alson, medical director of disaster services for the North Carolina Office of EMS. "You often have disparate groups who have individual issues, and having somebody who's neutral to guide the process can get you over some rocks and shoals."

## PROVIDER INVOLVEMENT AND ENGAGEMENT

At all of the regional workshops, as well as in the 2009 IOM report, one of greatest priorities identified was the need for extensive engagement with community and provider stakeholders. Provider stakeholders include not just doctors, nurses, EMTs, and other healthcare providers, but also participants in other parts of the healthcare system, including payers, regulators, the media, and the public. In a true public health emergency, each of these participants will have a critical role to play in achieving optimal care, and participants found uneven levels of understanding and commitment among these groups.

"About 3 years ago our quality management team put together a questionnaire just asking what one would do in the event of a pandemic flu outbreak," said Michael Spence of Kalispell Regional Medical Center, Montana. "From this, the ethics committee decided to develop a mass casualty group from the responses we got because we got various responses all over the map depending upon the type of person who was answering the questions."

Spence's group includes hospital leaders, epidemiologists, pharmacists, nurses, respiratory care technicians, emergency doctors, public health executives, hospital trustees, morticians, emergency services, and others. The group meets once a month and has worked with the local legislature to get laws passed facilitating the response to crisis standards of care.

### Engaging Frontline Providers

Spence wasn't the only one who found uneven preparations in the healthcare community. Despite all of the money and time spent on disaster preparedness, workshop participants observed that the penetration of that knowledge into the broader caregiver community is limited.

"The people who are hardest to get in the room and participate and speak are . . . the physicians," said Brian Currie, vice president and medical director for research at Montefiore Medical Center. "Most of the time they have to be chased to a meeting or have their arms bent to sit on a committee."

Several participants also expressed concern over the lack of involvement of emergency medical services (EMS) providers in the planning process. Frank Pratt, medical director of the Los Angeles County Fire

Department emphasized the importance of engaging EMS providers. "We are trapped [among] healthcare policy makers, elected officials, and citizens who are completely disconnected from the process" of planning for a disaster, said Pratt. "But we are the people who will be in someone's bedroom at 2:00 in the morning, making a decision."

One workshop participant cited a recent PricewaterhouseCoopers (PWC) report titled *Closing the Seams*. The report found that although $8 billion was spent on disaster preparedness since September 11, 2001, only 20 percent of the primary care providers surveyed believed they knew how to respond in a mass casualty situation (Pricewaterhouse-Coopers, 2007). That is compared to 100 percent of hospital executives, disaster coordinators, and public health departments. The PWC report highlights the fact that hospitals tend to operate in silos where personnel and information are not routinely shared. There is also no standard core of knowledge or credentialing regarding disaster preparedness.

The obvious answer to the problem is to regularly engage in training exercises. But given how stretched most doctors are already, getting them to take part in training exercises or think about disaster preparedness is nearly impossible, participants said. This was a rare corner of the topic in which there seemed to be few "best practices" from which to draw.

Asha Devereaux, a pulmonary and critical care physician in Coronado, CA, laid out some of the issues involved in engaging doctors in the issue of crisis standards of care (Box 9).

For most caregivers, however, a primary concern is time. Doctors and nurses are simply busy, working to save lives today, and do not have much time to plan for hypothetical disasters in the future.

---

**BOX 9**
**Engaging Doctors**

**Barriers to Understanding**

- Planning dollars spent on infrastructure and systems preparedness
- Silos of societies advocating their curriculum
- No time to prepare for rare event
- States and communities determine practice standards—more silos—but physicians receive education globally

---

**Potential Solution**

Educate physicians in language and venues in which they commonly receive information (avoid silos):
- Clear
- Concise
- Consensus based
- Clinical (most importantly)

Because of this, Peterson of the ANA noted that events such as the 2009 H1N1 virus must be seized as opportunities for on-the-job, real-world training. "The realities are in our day-to-day lives: Most nurses and other providers are busy . . . [and] the ability for them to take time off to really be able to engage in education . . . is very limited. How do we use teachable moments . . . as a way of engaging people in the conversation?"

A second issue is simply culture. Many workshop participants worried that physicians and nurses will resist the very concept of crisis standards of care, and will tend to push off the idea and assume that the resources will eventually be there. In a training scenario, you can remove those resources one by one until you arrive at a critical decision point. But convincing providers to actually face the reality of the situation could prove to be a major issue.

Then there are those who simply don't want to address the issues. "I hear providers . . . say 'Well, you know, if that's what I am going to be expected to do, I am sure as heck not showing up for work,'" noted Phillips. "Yes, someone has to do it, and I understand it is important, but it's not going to be me. That's not what I came into health care to do."

There were further concerns on how to engage doctors and caregivers outside the hospital setting. "Ambulatory physicians, infectious disease physicians [and others] have not really been at the table," said Currie. "How do you reach out and embrace people still practicing . . . anecdotal medicine . . . one patient, one problem, one process?"

One idea did rise to the top of the discussions: Pay providers to train. "I think we do what we're paid to do, and there are few financial incentives to exercise," said Shawn Rogers, director of EMS from the Oklahoma State Department of Health. Rogers went on to propose an innovative solution: "I think that if regular exercise participation was a condition of Medicare participation, we'd see a whole lot more of it." Cantrill of the Department of Emergency Medicine at Denver Health

Medical Center added that in order for that to be possible, the Centers for Medicare and Medicaid Services (CMS) would have to allow reimbursement for preparedness. He noted that this would be a critical step forward for hospital preparedness.

Even when training isn't possible, however, keeping providers in mind when designing the systems and methodologies will ensure more consistent implementation of crisis standards of care. When imagining a scenario that would require removing patients from life-sustaining care, Devereaux noted some of the following requirements: "We will need security to protect us from the demands of unrealistic family members. We will need transparency to assure us that other facilities are operating in the exact same manner. And we'll need constant communication and updates."

Others worried that, even with the best protocols, ensuring that doctors will follow through with the crisis standards remains a significant challenge. "When the rubber meets the road, when you have to make a decision to pull a patient off a vent, are we going to have individuals who are going to be willing to do that?" asked Cantrill. "I think it's a real challenge."

## Hospital Officials

For hospital officials, the reasons for not being engaged are similar— a lack of time, a lack of funding, and a concern about committing to rationed care—but the methodology for encouraging their commitment is different.

"All this discussion fits into the broader question of whether your business model will survive the next catastrophe," said Hanfling, putting himself in the administrator's shoes. "At the CEO [chief executive officer] level, they want to know that there is a revenue stream coming in after the fact. The reason we're looking at this is because we're talking about protecting our facilities, protecting our staff, providing an ongoing capability to our community-based mission."

Again, the opportunity for on-the-job training does present itself. Shawn Rogers, director of EMS for the Oklahoma State Department of Health and the President-Elect of the National Association of State EMS Officials, spoke of the experience of the Oklahoma City hospital groups, and how it took not one—but two—disasters to force executives to confront the need for a coordinated response:

[After the Oklahoma City bombing, there] was no system to share patients and appropriately distribute them. We, the medical community, in our after-action critique said, "[W]ell, we really need to do something about that" and then we didn't.

Four years later we had a big tornado and there were again centers where the tornado hit and there were lots of casualties and those hospitals nearby were again swarmed and the hospitals further out were not appropriately used. So we again had after-action reports and we got together and we said we really need to do something about that and we did.

We put together a metropolitan emergency resource center whose role was to coordinate where patients would go in disasters. The way we got the hospitals to buy into that was to ask for each hospital to send a representative to be trained and [be able to be activated] during a disaster. This representative would come down and man the resource center, one rep. from each hospital, to serve as the speaker to that facility in that disaster. The next time we had a tornado, in 2001, that hit down in the metro area and our response system worked rather well. Engaging facilities in that kind of a forum was effective for us.


## PUBLIC ENGAGEMENT AND EDUCATION

Many participants noted the importance of public engagement and education on this very difficult issue. If the public is not engaged in developing crisis standards of care, if it is not involved in evaluating the harsh choices that must be made, if it does not understand and agree with the ethics and logic surrounding those choices, even the best laid plans will fail.

"If you are going to alter how you deliver care, your public has to be on board," said the CDC's Levy. The public "will only follow [plans] if they (a) know about it and (b) have bought into it."

Melba Moore, commissioner of health from the City of St. Louis Department of Health, emphasized the importance of engaging the public. "You must be in the community. You must get out there because there is a history of distrust in the community of providers." Without that relationship no decision will get buy-in from the public.

Yet most workshop participants agreed this had not yet occurred.

"The public is . . . uneducated on this topic," said Brinsfield of DHS. "That's our fault because we're not sharing the information with them in a way that they can process and understand."

The question, though, is how to bring them into the discussion in an efficient, effective, and constructive way. Unfortunately, the easiest and most obvious approaches do not seem to work.

The Montefiore-Einstein Center's Powell noted that that bringing big community groups together to discuss these sorts of issues can be ineffective. "This is a really frightening issue, and if you're going to have 200 people together who have not spent their work lives contemplating this issue, it really slaps you in the face," she said. "You're going to have a couple of people who are really distressed in a not particularly productive way, and it can really derail that kind of meeting."

Powell recommended holding smaller focus group meetings, perhaps relying on community groups or faith-based organizations as a centralizing mechanism. Given how critical the public role could be in directing an emergency response, however, workshop participants explored two approaches, discussed in more detail below.

## Changing the Culture of Preparedness

The most comprehensive idea—and one which arose in multiple regional meetings and from multiple providers—was to use the heightened awareness after recent tragic events like Hurricane Katrina and September 11 to institute a new "culture of preparedness" in the community.

"I think one of the goals we as a group should have is to introduce preparedness into the national educational curriculum," suggested James Prudent, an emergency physician from New Jersey. "Just like patients come to us with something they've read online and compel us to go and learn about [new diseases] . . . if the public is energized to learn these things, then we too would be energized to learn these things."

Indeed, Shawn Fultz, senior medical advisor at the VHA, suggested creating a whole new culture around civil defense for the 21st century, an idea that was first broached during the Forum's March 2008 Workshop on Dispensing Medical Countermeasures (IOM, 2008). Just as children in the 1950s learned to "duck and cover," citizens today would learn how to respond to a bioterror attack, a pandemic flu, or a natural disaster.

It only takes a minute to realize how much a prepared population benefits the public health response. Models have suggested that a very large portion of the patients coming to the hospital during emergencies do not need urgent care. Preventing even half of these patients from clogging the system would free up tremendous resources. Similarly, having an informed public that understands that crisis standards of care are uniform across regional boundaries would discourage the inefficiencies and potential chaos that go along with "hospital shopping." Most importantly, an informed public should be better able to accept the sacrifices required in a mass casualty event, including understanding that resources may not exist to provide uninhibited care during the heart of the emergency.

"People are hungry for information," said Inova's Hanfling. "They're hungry for credible information that comes from trusted leaders."

If we can build a shared commitment and even a sense of civic responsibility, we will show the difference between panic and order, chaos and efficiency, and a population that works with the healthcare system during an emergency versus a population that revolts against the implementation of crisis standards of care.

"People are going to vote with their feet," noted Phillips. "How do we engage the public in this decision? [Some believe] we aren't really ready to engage the public yet because we haven't gotten our act together yet. But you could take it on the other side and say, well, if the public was part of getting our act together, then we wouldn't have to wait and then convey something to them."

The task of working with the public is a large one, and it's one for which users did not have a firm solution. Some even called for federal help. "I think it would be very useful from the federal level [to have a] tool kit that could be deployed regionally with health literacy, language barriers, and cultural competency . . . that could be modified per region . . . to address the specific cultural, spiritual, and community issues unique to our locals, but that would provide standardization in terms of the kind of information we are providing throughout the country," said Fleming.

## Elected Officials and the Media

The entity of the mass media is both a tremendous tool in a crisis and a significant challenge. The media will control the messages that most of a population receives in a crisis, and many workshop participants suggested that they should be assiduously courted as key stakeholders.

"It is critical to bring the media in early, because if they're in early and are a part of the planning process and see what goes into it, they're going to be much better prepared to support you during the time of disaster," said Nancy Auer, special medical advisor to the CEO at Swedish Medical Center in the state of Washington.

Workshop participants emphasized the importance of having a public information officer with the task of developing relationships with the media *before* a disaster strikes, so that those relationships can be leveraged after a disaster occurs. Others noted the importance of delivering a consistent message: Something simple, such as a universal agreement that the public should "shelter in place" and avoid the hospital unless they are truly critically ill, could prevent a wave of non-critically ill patients from besieging a facility.

"We had an approach in New York City . . . that we affectionately called 'One Voice,'" explained Walt Disney's Gabriel, who served previously as deputy commissioner for planning and preparedness for the New York City Office of Emergency Management.

The "One Voice" concept assumes that the public and the media will want to hear from a recognized leader—generally an elected official—during a disaster; think of then-Mayor Rudy Giuliani's role during the September 11 tragedy. That recognized leader may or may not be an expert on medical events, but if that leader is surrounded by the right people—legal counsel, hospital administrators, influential physicians, public health officials—and provided with consistent and reliable messaging, that "One Voice" will be able to drive forward the single message and inform the community of evolving standards.

This is the reason that efforts must be made to engage directly with elected officials and the media *before* events take place.

As with doctors, hospital administrators, and others, participants worried that elected leaders will blanch at the concept of implementing crisis standards of care.

## DEVELOPING INTRASTATE AND INTERSTATE COOPERATION AND CONSISTENCY

Without consistency across communities, regions, and states on crisis standards of care, there is much greater potential for chaos and unfairness. Participants at all of the workshops discussed the difficult balance between developing standards and procedures based on a community's particular values, characteristics, and needs, and ensuring a consistent approach across neighboring jurisdictions.

Different states have taken different approaches to developing crisis standards of care. Two that were highlighted at the meeting in New York were the approaches used by Massachusetts and Virginia. "Slightly different approach(s), though in reality our goals are similar," stated Lisa Kaplowitz, health director from the Alexandria Health Department in Virginia (Box 10).

"[Standards] should not be imposed from above," cautioned Powell of the Montefiore-Einstein Center. "But there does need to be a kind of crosschecking and a network of cooperation across the country so that plans are reasonably interchangeable, and there is an agreed-upon system or what people think are consistent and fair allocations of scarce resources."

Without consistent standards, patients will shop for hospitals with the most advantageous treatment protocols. Without consistency, individual physicians may be exposed to increased legal liability from patients who believe they could have received better care at a different hospital down the road. Without consistent standards and interneighbor cooperation, there cannot be a fair allocation of resources among neighboring facilities or by tapping into emergency reserves of supplies.

However, at each level of organization, from the departments of individual hospitals to communities, states, and regions, the issue becomes progressively more complicated. "If you think you have a problem trying to get adjacent hospitals to work together or communities to work together, imagine trying to do this across multiple states," said Terry Schenk, a consultant for the Florida Department of Health.

Several participants described existing mechanisms for interstate collaboration and cooperation that could serve as a basis for broad geographic coordination of crisis standards of care. In addition, consistency was a major theme of the IOM's letter report.

---

**BOX 10**
**Two States: Two Approaches**

**Massachusetts**

In 2006 The Commonwealth of Massachusetts convened a statewide committee to look at alternate care facilities. Initial and ongoing concerns were liability in a below-optimal resource environment and creating guidance that would help engender trust with the public. To that end:

- The committee developed various scenarios that dealt with issues such as limited care, providers' duty to come to work, the healthcare system's duty to providers in terms of protection, etc. and presented them to two focus groups, one made up of primarily physicians, and one primarily consumers.
- From the feedback and discussions in these groups, the committee is drafting statewide guidelines that (1) have ethical fundamental guidelines and (2) have a framework for implementing crisis standards of care.

SOURCES: Levin et al. (2009); The Commonwealth of Massachusetts Department of Public Health (2007).

**Virginia**

By contrast, the Commonwealth of Virginia's approach to crisis standards of care (or "care in situations of critical resource shortage," as Virginia calls it) is driven outside the umbrella of state government, instead delegating the planning authority to the medical community. To that end:

- A critical resource shortage guide was developed by a broad-based group from the Virginia Hospital and Healthcare Association.
- The guide helps the hospitals themselves "work through the process of how they're going to distribute resources when there is a critical shortage" as determined on the ground.

SOURCE: Virginia Department of Health (2008).

---

# FEMA Regions

A number of workshop participants highlighted the Federal Emergency Management Agency (FEMA) Emergency Response Regions as one way to subdivide the nation and create partnerships across state lines. FEMA divides the nation into 10 emergency response regions, each of which is tasked with protecting institutions from all types of hazards by developing a program to mitigate and respond to disaster scenarios. The regions have dedicated staff as well as on-call "reservists," who can be brought in to support regional response efforts.

The Region IV ESF-8 Unified Planning Coalition, bringing together representatives from Florida, Georgia, Kentucky, Mississippi, North Carolina, South Carolina, and Tennessee, received particular attention at the Orlando conference. "They have as their mission a collaborative effort to really look at . . . all hazards planning," added Terry Schenk, speaking of the same issue. "One of the things they are really trying to do is establish some consistency state to state."

James Blumenstock, chief program officer for public health practice at the Association of State and Territorial Health Officials said, "There are six or seven other regional coalitions around the country that exist primarily for the same purpose. . . . They have different levels of investments of leadership and they are really literally and figuratively all over the map with regards to the way they handle particular regional issues. I think that's a diamond in the rough for the purposes of building stronger regional coalition and coordination."

An obvious extension of this thinking, of course, is to create consistency from region to region. Disaster and diseases do not honor state lines or arbitrary regional designations. Blumenstock and others noted that, in an ideal scenario, regional and state-level planning committees would approach the problem of regional preparedness within a shared framework. This idea of regional and local coalitions operating under federal or other guidance was a theme that appeared again and again throughout the presentations.

## The All Hazards Consortium

In the National Capital Region (see http://www.ncrhomelandsecurity. org/), eight states have banded together to create an "All Hazards Consortium" that seeks to build collaboration to address the management of catastrophic events in and around the region. The states are Delaware, Maryland, New Jersey, New York, North Carolina, Pennsylvania, Virginia, and West Virginia. Their successes provide yet another model for approaching the problem.

As workshop participants noted, the states involved in the All Hazards Consortium secured a regional catastrophic planning grant from HHS. But rather than applying that grant to traditional planning exercises, it applied much of the money to developing a software system that will allow all of the emergency management organizations in those states to share information in real time. This software, updated and functioning, has been used for planning and training exercises, and stands ready to support event management and recovery the next time disaster strikes, explained Floyd Russell, Homeland Security liaison at the Office of the Vice President for Research and Economic Development at West Virginia University.

## The Interstate Disaster Medical Cooperative

The Interstate Disaster Medical Cooperative was created in 2007. The mission of the cooperative, as Timothy Conley, preparedness planning director at Western Springs Fire Department and Emergency Medical Services, IL, explained at the Chicago workshop, is to provide a forum to allow states to network with one another and share best practices. "The purpose of the interstate disaster medical cooperative is to establish for state medical teams a common framework and a way to work together," Conley said, "a way not to reinvent the wheel."

In addition to monthly teleconference calls and face-to-face meetings, the group is working together to create a standardized model of state operating procedures to promote interoperability and smooth the process whereby one group can surge to help another. The group also aims to identify both the special skills and the special resources housed in each state, to ensure a more robust regional response to specific emergencies. "Every state has a little bit of a different strength," said Conley, who noted that 20 states had signed up to participate in the cooperative.

The organization has created working groups to tackle specific issues, such as establishing and credentialing a Medical Reserve Corps or standardizing best practices for alternative care facilities. The group is also sponsoring a study on pediatric care during emergencies. In short, it is a grassroots organization tackling issue after issue in an effort to link people in an enhanced model of disaster preparedness.

## Village-to-Village Communication

Despite all the planning—and there is clearly a tremendous amount of solid groundwork being done—many participants worry that the boots-on-the-ground training has yet to start. There is a concern that, even where a regional system may be well fleshed out, local healthcare officials may be in the dark.

Conley brought up the example of his own town, the Village of Western Springs. When the H1N1 virus emerged, Western Springs developed an emergency response plan and laid out new protocols that took actions such as limiting provider interaction with the public to reduce illness; the neighboring town did nothing. Meanwhile, a third village in the area began requiring responders to wear masks on each EMS call. That level of confusion only served to foment panic in the public.

Conley also expressed serious concern that the local responders are not integrated into the planning taking place at the upper levels. "For the fun of it, I went out to one of the medics and asked them, 'Hey, what's our alternate care site for this region?' And guess what their answer was: They have no idea. They don't know that they won't be transporting cardiac arrest. They don't know that they will be making triage decisions whether somebody goes to a hospital or an alternate care site," Conley said.

Some level of just-in-time training on issues like this is surely inevitable: plans change, employees come and go, and training can never be totally universal. But the point is clear: planning cannot simply take place in the upper reaches of hospital departments, but must reach down to providers, emergency medical service providers, homecare nurses, and other critical points on the healthcare chain.


## Communications and Consistency

Communications among stakeholders during an emergency was a critical issue that was mentioned throughout the meetings, with different groups taking different approaches. Sometimes, the solution is as simple as having the right phone system in place.

Chris Dent, an infection prevention nurse at Saint Alphonsus Regional Medical Center in Idaho, told the Irvine workshop about the work that the Idaho Hospital Coalition had done to set up a "bridge call service." The service allows emergency management systems to contact area hospitals, who are then required to dial into a shared conference-call number. That shared conference call serves as a confidential and reliable source on the exact nature of an emergency and the plans regarding interfacility cooperation, supply sharing, and standards of care.

"The bridge calls [let us] tell the hospitals what the real story is, not what gossip is coming in over the radio," noted Dent. "We have not only practiced this, but have used it . . . including during a vaccine shortage. We used the bridge call to come up with [a plan] so that every hospital was using vaccines in the same way."

Although no system will foresee every eventuality or forecast every concern, establishing lines of communication in advance can improve the application of consistent crisis standards of care during an emergency. At the workshop in Florida, Lori Upton, assistant director of emergency management at Texas Children's Hospital, described the circumstances that led to increased coordination and communication among stakeholders in her region (Box 11).

---

**BOX 11**
**A Lesson Learned**

"Back in 2001," said Lori Upton, assistant director of emergency management for Texas Children's Hospital, "before the collapse of the World Trade Center, we had a little storm that came over Houston called Allison. It dropped 34 inches of rain on us and it completely wiped out the Texas Medical Center in downtown Houston . . . which includes 13 large facilities with medical schools attached to it. So we wiped out over 5,000 hospital beds in one evening, and it was Labor Day weekend.

We learned about evacuations of health care. We learned about alternate standards of care for patients that were leaving an acute care facility and going to an alternate care site or going to a nursing home because they were stable and the nursing homes had beds. What we didn't have at the time is we didn't have a coordinating entity: one person or one voice that was able to get all of the information out to the hospitals to let them know what's happening, what the standards are right now, and who's going where, and who's going to be moving when.

As a result, we formed a regional hospital-preparedness council . . . and now it includes every hospital in the region. It includes our EMS providers, our ME's offices, our VA and EMS liaisons, our offices of emergency management, our public health, medical societies, our nursing schools, our medical schools . . . all of our partners that we may touch. They come together once a month.

. . . We [now] have a catastrophic medical operations center that falls underneath our public health authority. We have one coordinating entity that our hospitals look for, EMS look for regarding transportation, for asset utilization, etc."

## THE ROLE OF THE FEDERAL GOVERNMENT AND NATIONAL LEADERSHIP

The role of the federal government in helping to guide and facilitate the development of crisis standards of care was highly debated at the workshops. Some participants worried that a heavy-handed approach from Washington could derail more in-the-trenches attempts to develop plans at the state and local levels and lead to policies that are inconsistent with state and local values and needs. Many participants, however, believed some level of guidance at the federal or national level would be helpful. They saw a range of ways that federal or national leadership could facilitate the development of fair and consistent crisis standards of care policies and protocols, and could help reduce unnecessary duplication of effort.

On the practical end, there was a widespread call for the federal government to perform a role as "chief information coordinator" on the topic of crisis standards of care. "There are people all across the country and states, at county and other facility levels, who really are kind of reinventing the wheel," said Montefiore's Powell. They are "starting all over again, trying to do the literature search and figure out what's going on. It's an enormous investment of time and manpower across the country when in fact there are scholars who at least have some of that information as ready knowledge."

Indeed, that insight was demonstrated tangibly at the workshops, where dozens of state and local plans were presented, each of which required huge investments of time and energy to produce, and each of which in many cases ended up with similar conclusions. If a way to index that information in a single location as a resource was established, Powell and others suggested, it would massively improve the efficiency of developing these guidelines throughout the nation.

Federal or national involvement would also provide a level of legal, societal, and practical protection that cannot be achieved at the lower levels of leadership. Many people at the workshops noted that there may be some issues for which federal or national involvement is the only practical choice.

"These are politically explosive issues," noted Powell. "At every single facility and even at the state level you'll have people who either don't want to talk about it or just come up with vague guidelines . . . because it's a liability risk." What's needed, she suggested, is an acknowledgment at the highest level that the issue is worth talking about, and that the uncomfortable must be confronted. "I think the higher you come from in saying that, the more security there is in believing that will be an acceptable plan."

Looking at the bigger picture, participants noted that having broad federal guidance could help establish consistency from state to state and region to region. The unfortunate reality is that anything other than national guidance risks running into "border issues" in areas where one region, state, or community butts up against another. A coordinating policy that bridges those gaps and establishes a framework of consistency would be immensely valuable.

Many workshop participants praised the aforementioned work of AHRQ and ASPR to establish the outlines of a framework in their 2005 report, *Altered Standards of Care in Mass Casualty Events* and 2007 report, *Mass Medical Care with Scarce Resources: A Community Planning Guide* (AHRQ, 2005; Phillips and Knebel, 2007). These documents, however, only go as far as making broad recommendations about the scope and challenges that should be considered and laying out preliminary implementation considerations. Many workshop participants wanted more.

"We've got to start identifying players and start trying to get to some specificity of what that national guidance could look like," said the ANA's Peterson. She added that establishing evidence-based research for making decisions about crisis standards of care represents a massive and immediate opportunity for a nationally convening organization. Much of the work on crisis standards of care and emergency response is driven by principles and best guesses; there is little existing evidence about what works and what doesn't in various situations.

These knowledge gaps extend from treatment protocols to triage to equipment usage. For example, there is little evidence about the use of SOFA scores for predicting outcomes in pediatric or geriatric populations, or about which simple treatments achieve the best outcome at acute care facilities during a pandemic influenza.

All of those things can be known to some extent using historical data on past tragedies or studies in non-disaster scenarios. But the unfortunate reality is that there has been neither the funding nor the initiative to do much direct, evidence-based disaster medical research.

One thing was clear from the workshops: Most participants did not want the federal government dictating the specifics of how to *implement* policies.

"One can't get too prescriptive on the actual protocols, for a couple of reasons," said Kristi Koenig, director of public health preparedness at University of California–Irvine. "One, the solutions are going to vary from community to community. And two, a lot of these are evolving situations, where resources are coming in and getting more scarce throughout."

But still, the opportunity for the federal government to establish broad principles, roles, and objectives, as it did in a strong first step in the AHRQ documents—and then to take that one step forward by serving as a convening mechanism and research coordinator for multiple parties—is evident. Workshop participants suggested the time is now.

"In the context of the broader picture of healthcare reform, and with a shift in the administration . . . I'd like to see leadership from the top really help to bring this forward now . . . on a national level," said Inova's Hanfling.

Workshop participants' call for federal and national leadership to provide practical, more detailed information to advance the development of crisis standards of care protocols, and to facilitate intrastate and interstate consistency, formed the basis for the subsequent Institute of Medicine committee report entitled *Guidance for Establishing Crisis Standards of Care for Use in Disaster Situations* (IOM, 2009). This letter report, summarized in Appendix B, provides guidance on ethical considerations; community and provider engagement, education, and communication; legal authority and environment; indicators and triggers; and clinical process and operations. The committee calls on states to work to ensure consistency in the implementation of crisis standards of care throughout the state and among neighboring states.


## The Veterans Health Administration

The VHA was mentioned by a number of participants as both an untapped resource for support during emergencies and an underused resource for planning national, regional, and neighborhood collaboration.

The VHA runs more than 150 hospitals and some 800 outpatient medical clinics around the country, as well as 200-plus "Veterans Centers." At each regional meeting, VHA representatives made a point of stating that they would be available—in most scenarios—as a resource for the community during disasters.

"We have a requirement to support both internal and external missions," said Richard Callis, deputy chief consultant for planning and operations at the VHA. "We also have a responsibility under the emergency management support function . . . that requires working throughout the VHA system to bring clinicians to support field operations" during a disaster.

Several participants reiterated that the VHA actually has staff with full-time responsibilities for disaster preparedness, fulfilling a statutory mission for emergency management not just for the VHA system, but throughout the whole community. "There is one person assigned as the regional emergency manager for each FEMA region," noted Fultz of the VHA. He added that these employees oversee additional staff.

The VHA representatives at the workshops suggested that communities looking to develop standardized supply and response tactics should tap into this VHA network aggressively. While it operates in multiple regions and hundreds of communities, it is also a single, national, integrated system. Therefore, several workshop participants suggested, it represents a unique opportunity to facilitate the development of consistent crisis standards of care across the nation. The IOM letter report also reached this conclusion (IOM, 2009).

## The Department of Defense

One other way that the federal government can lead, many said, is by leveraging its position as a large provider and purchaser of healthcare services. That leadership can come through direct purchasing power; as noted earlier, some believe that provider participation in the Medicare program should be predicated on adequate disaster preparedness and emergency management training. Or it can come from serving as a model for other regions or localities in how to develop crisis standards of care. Wayne Hachey, director of preventive medicine for the Office of the Assistant Secretary of Defense, presented at the Irvine and Orlando workshops.

The Department of Defense is "the largest federal agency with a healthcare system," Hachey said. "Throughout our DoD guidance, we've recognized that we will have to establish alternate standards of care [during an emergency] . . . and those standards of care will not be consistent with today's standard."

"We don't have a DoD-wide standard," Hachey explained. "What we've told folks is that their standards are going to mirror, at least as a baseline, the standards of the civilian community."

In other words, the DoD program recognizes that each DoD facility has different staffing, different physical plans, a different population to serve, and different equipment and resources. So rather than forcing a top-down standard, it gives hospital administrators the opportunity to adapt their existing standards to the situation at hand. The only caveat, mentioned above, is that those standards be at or above the level of the surrounding community (Box 12). "Rather than being prescriptive, we gave them essentially rules of engagement in establishing altered standards of care," said Hachey.

To help create and monitor those standards, each installation within the DoD has a Public Health Emergency Officer with responsibility for advising the station commander during a significant public health emergency. This officer also coordinates with the local community to ensure the military and civilian response plans are integrated. Again, the IOM letter report called on state and local officials to coordinate with DoD facilities in the development and implementation of their standards of care protocols (IOM, 2009).

"When we developed guidelines for prioritizing care . . . the request from our providers [was] asking for both prescriptive guidance but probably more importantly [was asking] for permission to make those kinds of decisions," Hachey said. "So we gave them broad guidance, gave them sanction, made sure that they made their decisions transparent . . . [and] mandated that their standards of care at least as baseline be the same as their local standards of care."

---

**BOX 12**
**Department of Defense Resource Prioritization Policy**

- Crisis Standards of Care will be adopted—those standards will be locally determined based on resources, demographics, and prioritization principles
- It will not close its doors to the beneficiary population—those enrolled for care at Military Treatment Facilities will continue to get care at that facility unless guaranteed elsewhere BEFORE the pandemic
- Baseline standard of care will be comparable to local civilian standards
- Some Department of Defense personnel will receive medical resources above the standard of care despite lower medical risk due to operational requirements
- Mandates transparency BEFORE the emergency

## ETHICAL CONSIDERATIONS

The ethical issues in situations with scarce resources and crisis standards are both challenging and fundamental. They are challenging, as one workshop participant put it, because they contradict many of the values we hold dearest, such as providing each patient with the best available care.

But the ethical issues raised by these questions are fundamental for other reasons. They are fundamental because if we don't act in accordance with our ethical principles, the repercussions both for individuals and the society after the fact will be enormous. They are fundamental because our ethical principles serve as the foundation of our laws. They are fundamental because people will only act and sacrifice if they believe they are operating in an ethical system, and that individuals are being treated with fairness and transparency in the full view of the law. In addition, they are fundamental, quite frankly, because many of the decisions contemplated will be made with imperfect information—they will be best guesses. Those guesses, in the absence of firm evidence, will need to be made based on a shared ethical construct.

As the workshops revealed, the work done on crisis standards of care focuses a great deal on achieving consistency, in part because consistency and fairness are integral to any ethical system. The 2009 IOM letter report outlines seven ethical considerations that are central to the development of ethical crisis standards of care protocols: fairness, duty to care, duty to steward resources, transparency, proportionality, and accountability (IOM, 2009). However, applying the ethical framework is difficult because these are challenging questions that rarely have obvious, singular "right" answers.

Powell of the Montefiore-Einstein Center presented the work her committee did when establishing an ethical framework for ventilator allocation during public health emergencies in New York (Powell et al., 2008). One question that came up immediately in the discussions, she said, was whether healthcare workers would receive priority access to ventilators during an emergency.

The points in favor of such a policy are obvious: Healthcare workers take extra risks during public health emergencies, especially in infectious situations such as a pandemic flu. If they are not given priority access to care, some may not show up to work. If healthcare workers don't show up to work, fewer people will get care. It is a logical, reasoned argument for granting those workers priority access.

On the flipside, Powell noted, plenty of people take risks. Those include non-physicians inside and outside the hospital, such as custodians, nurses, respiratory techs, EMTs, and more. "You include all those people, and if your crisis is bad enough, I think you just ran out of ventilators and nobody in your community has them, only the healthcare workers." Moreover, said Powell, if a ventilator triage program is structured based on employment, children are excluded.

A continuing question is that of priority, Powell added. Too often, she suggested, the people who write the rules for priority access put themselves at the top of the list. She cited one case where the rules were drawn up by a legislating body, and somehow, elected officials ended up at the top of the list.

The problem, of course, is that arguments can be made for many different constituencies. As a general rule, if the people making the prioritization list end up at the top, the community is unlikely to buy in to the program.

For the New York standard, Powell's group decided that access to ventilators would be based solely on medical evaluations. Rather than granting healthcare workers priority access, New York decided to do more to protect them from getting sick in the first place.

It's important to note that Powell wasn't necessarily positioning New York's decision as "the right one." But it was "a right one" because it reflected the considered values of the community.

Many workshop participants stressed the importance of community values and the need to involve communities in the ethical planning process before a crisis hits.

Fortunately, as the workshops revealed, there is a tremendous trove of research that can be tapped into regarding the ethical issues surrounding crisis standards of care, including the work by Powell and many others (DeBruin et al., 2009; IOM, 2009; Powell et al., 2008; VHA, 2009a). Tools, guidebooks, and online planning systems can help communities walk through the process of developing ethically sound crisis standards of care (New Jersey Hospital Association, 2008; VHA, 2008b). One tool that multiple users pointed to was the IntegratedEthics tool offered on the website of the VHA's National Center for Ethics in Health Care (VHA, 2009b). Developed by leading experts in the field and tested in a number of scenarios, it was highly recommended as a good starting point for communities.

But this work needs to be done before disasters strike. In the heat of the battle, there won't be time to raise community awareness or think through the ethical implications of each answer. That can put caregivers into impossible situations with extraordinary potential repercussions.

"You need to be able to give your workers at least one right answer," said Powell. "It's true that there's not only one right answer, but [you don't want to] make them do the wrong thing." More work is needed on allocation of scarce resources, workforce issues, community involvement, and consistency.

Either way, ethical requirements come first, and must be integrated from the beginning.

## LEGAL ISSUES FOR CRISIS STANDARDS OF CARE

Legal concerns hover over every issue in disaster planning and crisis standards of care. "Laws absolutely pervade emergency responses at every level of the government," explained James Hodge, then executive director at Johns Hopkins' Center for Law and the Public's Health, one of several legal experts who presented at the four regional workshops. "Laws determine what constitutes a public health or other type of emergency; they help create the infrastructure through which we respond, prevent, and detect these emergencies; they authorize the performance or non-performance of various different actions by a host of different actors; and they flat-out determine the extent of responsibility for potential or actual harms that arise during emergencies."

Planning ahead to ensure that the legal environment will support an effective, fair, and consistent response is a crucial step in preparing for crisis standards of care during an emergency event. Workshop participants found that this area still needs a significant amount of work.

### Legal Liability

Most states have provisions that limit legal liability during emergencies. Ball from South Carolina outlined a number of laws that help limit medical malpractice liability during emergency situations in South Carolina, including the following:

- *Emergency Health Powers Act* (44-5-570, (C)(1)): "Any health care provider appointed by [the South Carolina Department of Health & Environmental Control] . . . must not be held liable for civil damages as a result of medical care . . . unless the damages result from . . . circumstances demonstrating a reckless disregard for the consequences."

- *Medical Malpractice Act* (38-79-30): "Volunteer (non-compensated) health care provider . . . not liable for any civil damage for any act or omission resulting from the rendering of the (medical) services unless . . . act or omission was the result of . . . gross negligence or willful misconduct."

Similar laws exist in most other states. But although these laws represent a good start, they come with one major drawback during crisis standards situations. Raymond Pepe of the Uniform Law Commission (ULC) noted that the laws "by and large immunize ordinary acts of negligence while not immunizing gross negligence or willful disregard of standards of care." Despite the drawbacks of this limitation, several participants added, it is also necessary to discourage harmful behavior and protect patients from those who do not act in good faith during disaster responses.

Crisis standards contemplated include not offering or discontinuing life-sustaining treatments such as ventilators as part of a broader triage program. "When we willfully and knowingly withdraw or withhold life support, knowing there may be a bad outcome, we tread that line of willful misconduct," said Cheryl Starling of the California Department of Public Health. Starling and others noted that this is one of the key barriers to getting healthcare providers and facilities to come to the table to discuss crisis standards of care and disaster preparedness.

These issues, she said, make "lawyers run for the hills and refuse to let people even talk about this . . . because [many people believe] you're setting yourself up for negligence and willful misconduct." This fear is especially strong with regard to the most extreme situations that involve the need to discontinue life-sustaining treatment in some patients.

These issues can also make healthcare providers unwilling to act during these emergencies, even with the clearest directions in place by top-level public health administrators. If you can't solve the legal liability issue, many noted, you can't get anywhere.

Fortunately, a great deal of work has been done on this issue at both the federal and state levels, creating a reference body of potential options for various localities to explore.

*Addressing the Liability Problem*

The first question that must be asked when approaching the problem of legal liability, Pepe said, is what legal liability is based on. "An accepted community standard of care grows out of either custom or practice, or it grows out of outcomes-based research which has led to consensus with respect to how to treat certain conditions," said Pepe. "When you're dealing with an alternative standard of care, you're dealing with something fundamentally different. There's a need to have clear legal recognition that these alternative standards exist and that practitioners are authorized to follow them."

It is important to note that there is a critical distinction between legal and medical standards of care (Box 13). Starling noted that the term "standard of care" actually comes from a legal setting, not a medical setting, defining the duty to provide a minimum acceptable standard of care. "The medical standard of care may be higher than that, but defining the legal bare-minimum of that standard of care . . . and analyzing how that will change during emergencies . . . is a critical issue that requires more work," Starling said.

Participants discussed a variety of ways in which the actual legal protections could be achieved.

---

**BOX 13**
**Medical and Legal Standards of Care**

**Medical Standards of Care:** The type and level of medical care required in specific circumstances by professional norms, accreditation or other requirements.

**Legal Standards of Care:** The amount of skill that a medical practitioner should exercise in particular circumstances based on reasonable and common practice in medical care.

---

*Deputize Physicians*

James Geiling, chief of medical services at the White River Junction VA Medical Center, VT, noted that some states have simply "deputized" physicians during states of emergency, or the federal government can make them federal agents. These actions can be enacted rapidly, and those deputized as state agents receive the state's "sovereign immunity-type protections" that exist in many jurisdictions.

The complication of this action is that these deputized workers become the legal agents of the state or the federal government, and they must therefore be prepared to perform as the state or federal government mandates, not necessarily what their own healthcare institution or other usual employer might require. That concept can make many healthcare institutions and employers very uncertain, and they may be unwilling to cede that control.

*Enact Comprehensive Liability Protection*

Other states have taken more nuanced approaches. Virginia has enacted a comprehensive liability protection program that goes into effect if there is a declaration of emergency on behalf of the state government and it has resulted in resource shortages. Critically, the Virginia law does not require a separate act by the legislature to go into effect, but can be put into effect by the governor's credo.

Montana passed a bill earlier in 2009 "that very much touches altered standards of care in an emergent situation if declared by the governor and protects us and gives us some immunity—and it's different from the code of practice that we have," noted Orlando meeting participant Michael Spence of Kalispell Regional Medical Center, MT.

A theme throughout the workshops was the concept of moving up the political chain of command when empowering this kind of legal liability protection, and putting the declaration of the emergency in the hands of a single powerful individual, such as a governor. Colorado, for instance, has draft executive orders that the governor can enact and that provide blanket protections for everything from license issues to who can dispense medicine.

Finding ways to make the standards as consistent and evenly applied as possible will be critical to mitigating liability for providers who are trying to do the right thing. That means, for example, having liability protections that extend not just to doctors and nurses, but to triage officers, resource teams, and all other parties involved in the healthcare process. Persons involved in triage were of particular concern because triage is where many of the most difficult decisions must be made. Participants mentioned the challenge and importance of developing consistency across state lines, and this was also a theme in the 2009 IOM letter report (IOM, 2009).

## Credentialing and Scope of Practice

In contemplating the legal ramifications of enacting crisis standards of care, one issue that was raised repeatedly at the workshops was the credentialing of out-of-state healthcare providers. Other means of augmenting the core caregiver community were seen as critical, including expanding the types of care that certain healthcare providers can provide and supporting retired healthcare workers who are interested in volunteering during times of crisis.

Participants discussed the critical importance of having sufficient, qualified personnel during an emergency. Finding ways to expand the size and scope of the caregiver community, while maintaining and supporting a community-based vision for crisis standards of care, was seen as a critical task.

One group that has taken the lead on this work is the Uniform Law Commission, an interstate organization that has done extensive work on the credentialing issue and has developed a draft law—the *Uniform Emergency Volunteer Health Practitioners Act*—that states can adopt (Box 14). It includes a robust system for the interstate recognition of healthcare licenses.

"It takes the fundamental approach that there is no reason that if your state is affected by a disaster you need to review on a case-by-case basis the credentials of people who are coming in from other states," said the ULC's Pepe.

The law limits the scope of medicine that these outside practitioners can practice, but it takes a common-sense approach of smoothing their entry into the disaster response. The idea is that multiple states can adopt the law in its written format.

---

**BOX 14**
**Uniform Emergency Volunteer Health Practitioners Act**

- Helps remove some of the barriers to implementing alternative standards of care
- Provides a model for promoting interstate cooperation
- Avoids the need for federal preemption
- Robust system for interstate recognition of health practitioner licenses (supplements the Emergency Management Assistance Compact)
- Extends civil immunity and workers compensation benefits to emergency volunteers
- Defines permissible interstate scope of practice
- Permits modifications to scope of practice
- Enhances state emergency management authority
- Controls spontaneous volunteerism
- Creates interstate system for disciplinary enforcement

---

At the same time, statutes across the country envision expanding scopes of practice temporarily for existing healthcare providers to let them work beyond the boundaries of their traditional expertise. Pharmacists may be asked to administer vaccinations, nurses may be asked to function in the role of nurse practitioners, and emergency medical technicians may be asked to dispense medicine.

Similarly, many states have statutes that allow retired healthcare providers to provide a limited set of services, such as palliative care. These healthcare providers can be a tremendous aid during an emergency, many noted, as long as they are given tasks appropriate to their training and education.

"We polled about 10,000 different perspective volunteers back in 2006," said Johns Hopkins' Hodge. "Seventy percent of them, or nearly 70 percent, said that their potential exposure to liability is an important or essential fact in whether or not they'll actually participate in an emergency."

The math is simple: Better, clearer legal protections mean more personnel to confront a mass casualty event.


## EMTALA and HIPAA

Multiple workshop participants expressed concerns about the impact of federal regulations—specifically, the *Emergency Medical Treatment and Labor Act* (EMTALA) and the *Health Insurance Portability and Accountability Act* (HIPAA)—on the ability to respond to a medical disaster (Box 15). EMTALA requires certain hospitals to provide emergency care to all patients, regardless of their ability to pay; patients may not simply be denied care and turned away from the hospital's doors. HIPAA governs privacy regulations and restricts the sharing of medical information. Compliance with these regulations is a significant concern for hospitals because failure to comply can result in exclusion from the Medicare program.

"How are you going to triage people to . . . alternate sites when you have EMTALA regulations in your face?" asked one participant, capturing the concerns of many. "How are you going to transfer people to other facilities when you have HIPAA that's not going to let you get information back?"

To some extent, these specific concerns are already accounted for in the existing legal system. An apparently less well-known fact about the HIPAA and EMTALA regulations is that, when the HHS Secretary declares a public health emergency and the President declares an emergency or a disaster pursuant to the *National Emergencies Act* or the *Stafford Act*, HHS can issue an "1135 waiver" that temporarily suspends sanctions for noncompliance with certain provisions under both HIPAA and EMTALA.[2] These waivers have been enacted in the past, and can be put in place quickly (and retroactively) during a disaster setting.

---

**BOX 15**
**EMTALA and HIPAA**

**EMTALA:** The ***Emergency Medical Treatment and Labor Act*** was enacted by Congress in 1986 to "ensure public access to emergency services regardless of ability to pay." The law requires hospitals participating in the Medicare system to provide medical screening examinations to patients requesting treatment for emergency medical conditions. Hospitals must also provide stabilizing treatment for these conditions, or, if such treatment is outside the hospital's capability, provide an appropriate transfer (http://www.cms.hhs.gov/emtala/).

**HIPAA:** Enacted by Congress in 1996, the ***Health Insurance Portability and Accountability Act*** protects the privacy of a patient's personal health information. Medical providers are allowed to disclose that information "for patient care and other important purposes" (http://www.hhs.gov/ocr/privacy/hipaa/understanding/index.html).

---

[2] See http://www.ssa.gov/OP_Home/ssact/title11/1135.htm.

Florida's Hood, however, cautioned about taking this comfort too far, noting that "many states have laws about medical confidentiality which are stricter than HIPAA."

Hood and others noted that the 1135 waivers do not impact these more restrictive state-level laws. The recommendation was that states should individually evaluate their laws and put in place emergency orders to remove barriers to emergency response.

## Legal Triage

Regardless of what legal rules are in place, or what standards have been agreed to, the legal landscape will be constantly shifting during an emergency, and participants will likely have to adjust their response accordingly.

Johns Hopkins' Hodge introduced his own concept of "legal triage" to define how healthcare administrators must constantly adjust their operating procedures throughout an emergency to remain consistent with the evolving situation (Hodge and Anderson, 2008; Hodge et al., 2009). "It's about prioritizing . . . legal issues in real time to construct a favorable legal environment . . . that facilitates legitimate public health responses during emergencies," said Hodge. "Once an emergency has been declared, by design the legal landscape changes. . . . [I]t changes instantly and it can change drastically, and depending on how it changes, based on the type of emergency that we're involved with, the legal responsibilities and liability protections and altered standards of care issues come into play."

Hodge noted that since September 11, 2001, many new laws have been put into place governing emergency response and disaster preparedness. Forty-two states now officially allow for a declaration of disaster, and 26 states specifically define a public health emergency. The peculiarities of how those disasters are declared and what the term "disaster" actually means, legally, varies in nearly every case. Quite often there are different levels of declaration. "Your deployment, your abilities, your authorities, your liabilities, immunities are all dependent upon that level of an emergency," explained Hodge.

In the midst of a disaster, having a legal team in place that is ready to respond to and interpret those evolving legal standards can be just as important as having the right medical triage and response teams. The message throughout the meetings was that if communities did not take care of the legal issues, much of the other planning would be significantly less effective.

## Education and Training

As well-designed and thoughtful as any legal liability protections or other crisis standards laws may be, their effectiveness rests on whether hospital administrators and their legal counsel know they exist.

A theme that emerged from the legal discussions was that the natural reaction at many hospitals is to protect against liability and limit activity, barring clear guidance otherwise. That will likely be the prevailing wisdom in the confusion sure to accompany a true healthcare disaster.

Workshop participants repeatedly observed that significant work was needed to disseminate information about legal liability protections to healthcare providers, even in those states that have tackled the problem head-on.

## CONCLUSION

How can healthcare providers and facilities, with the support of state and local public health officials, the federal government, and their communities, provide the best care possible during a crisis? What steps can the health system take to avoid resource scarcity, manage demand, and minimize impact on clinical care? If these steps become insufficient, how should resources be allocated fairly and consistently? How can these steps be taken in an ethical, legal, and effective manner?

These were the questions that knitted together the four regional workshops in California, Florida, New York, and Illinois. While the individual approaches varied, participants were unified in recognizing that these were important questions, and that they were questions that had to be answered before it was too late.

A great deal of progress has been made over the past decade, motivated in part by events such as September 11, 2001, the anthrax attacks, and Hurricane Katrina. Ten years ago, hospital administrators and healthcare officials wouldn't touch the third rail of crisis standards of care; now working groups are approaching this problem in regions, states, and communities around the nation. The workshops presented dozens of approaches, many of which shared common basic principles, even if they differed on the specifics. National efforts from the CDC, AHRQ, and others were widely praised for laying the groundwork, even as participants identified more work that needs to be done.

These are not easy issues. The scenarios addressed at these meetings are uncomfortable. Fearsome words like "rationing" and dire concepts like discontinuing life-sustaining treatment in critically ill patients must be considered and confronted head-on, at every level—from federal oversight to local administrations—and by every party—from politicians to lawyers to primary caregivers.

Ultimately, the discussions are held with the aim of providing the best and most fair treatment to as many patients as possible during a crisis.

Healthcare providers will not have time during an emergency to develop programs from a standpoint of fairness and equity. There will not be time to develop laws to facilitate information sharing, dramatically increase staff, or provide legal liability. Any on-the-spot efforts to develop triage protocols, conduct evidence-based studies, or build relationships of trust among hospitals in different regions and communities will be impossible.

As a result, participants said, officials have a duty to plan for these scenarios. They have a duty to develop crisis standards of care protocols based on reasoned and ethical approaches that reflect the views and beliefs of the broader community. While much has been done, that work needs to be gathered into a central resource where other jurisdictions can reference and use it, and more evidence-based research is needed. Importantly, more work needs to be done to build relationships and ensure consistency in the approach of different regions and settings.

But there is more work to do, especially in some areas that will be critical during crises:

- Palliative care planning: Caregivers and administrators need everything from simple definitions to detailed guidance on when and where it is given and who can provide it.
- Mental/behavioral health implications for the public as well as care providers.
- Preparedness planning for vulnerable populations, such as pediatric, geriatric, and mental health patients.
- Public and provider engagement in the planning process.
- Consistency across borders and regions.

"How far do we need to get in standards?" asked Phillips, summarizing the Irvine meeting. "Are they general principles that we should all be adhering to? Do we need to be setting some national standards? Should we be just aiming toward principles that ensure consistency, but allowing individual flexibility?"

Overall, participants said that the workshops had been helpful in highlighting how much work is going on around the nation on this issue, but also emphasized that much work remains to be done in order to ensure that the best care possible is provided under catastrophic circumstances.

# A

# References

AHRQ (Agency for Healthcare Research and Quality). 2005. *Altered standards of care in mass casualty events.* AHRQ Publication No. 05-0043. Rockville, MD: AHRQ.

ANA (American Nurses Association). 2008. *Adapting standards of care under extreme conditions: Guidance for professionals during disasters, pandemics, and other extreme emergencies.* http://www.nursing world.org/MainMenuCategories/HealthcareandPolicyIssues/DPR/TheLaw EthicsofDisasterResponse/AdaptingStandardsofCare.aspx (accessed September 8, 2009).

California Department of Public Health. 2008. *Standards and guidelines for healthcare surge during emergencies.* http://bepreparedcalifornia. ca.gov/EPO/CDPHPrograms/PublicHealthPrograms/EmergencyPrepared nessOffice/EPOProgramsServices/Surge/StandGuide/SSG1.htm (accessed September 8, 2009).

CMS (Centers for Medicare and Medicaid Services). 2002. *MDS 2.0 for nursing homes.* http://www.cms.hhs.gov/nursinghomequalityinits/20_NHQIMDS 20.asp (accessed September 9, 2009).

Colorado Department of Public Health and Environment. 2009 (unpublished). *Guidance for alterations in the healthcare system during a moderate to severe influenza pandemic.*

DeBruin, D., E. Parilla, J. Liaschenko, M. Marshall, J. Leider, D. Brunnquell, J. Garrett, and D. Vawter. 2009. *Implementing ethical frameworks for rationing scarce health resources in Minnesota during severe influenza pandemic: Preliminary report.* http://www.ahc.umn.edu/mnpanflu/prod/ groups/ahc/@pub/@ahc/@ethicsmpep/documents/content/ahc_content_090 510.pdf (accessed September 9, 2009).

Devereaux, A. V., J. R. Dichter, M. D. Christian, N. N. Dubler, C. E. Sandrock, J. L. Hick, T. Powell, J. A. Geiling, D. E. Amundson, T. E. Baudendistel, D. A. Braner, M. A. Klein, K. A. Berkowitz, J. R. Curtis, and L. Rubinson. 2008. Definitive care for the critically ill during a disaster: A framework for allocation of scarce resources in mass critical care: From a Task Force for Mass Critical Care Summit meeting, January 26–27, 2007, Chicago, IL. *Chest* 133(5 Suppl):51S–66S.

Flacker, J. M., and D. K. Kiely. 1998. A practical approach to identifying mortality-related factors in established long-term care residents. *J Am Geriatr Soc* 46(8):1012–1015.

Gebbie, K. M., C. A. Peterson, I. Subbarao, and K. M. White. 2009. Adapting standards of care under extreme conditions. *Disaster Med Public Health Prep* 3(2):111–116.

Hick, J. L., and D. T. O'Laughlin. 2006. Concept of operations for triage of mechanical ventilation in an epidemic. *Acad Emerg Med* 13(2):223–229.

Hick, J. L., J. A. Barbera, and G. D. Kelen. 2009. Refining surge capacity: Conventional, contingency, and crisis capacity. *Disaster Med Public Health Prep* 3(2 Suppl):S59–S67.

Hodge, J., and E. Anderson. 2008. Principles and practice of legal triage during public health emergencies. *NYU Annual Survey of American Law* 64:249–292.

Hodge, J. G., Jr., A. M. Garcia, E. D. Anderson, and T. Kaufman. 2009. Emergency legal preparedness for hospitals and health care personnel. *Disaster Med Public Health Prep* 3(2 Suppl):S37–S44.

IOM (Institute of Medicine). 2008. *Dispensing medical countermeasures for public health emergencies: Workshop summary.* Washington, DC: The National Academies Press.

IOM. 2009. *Guidance for establishing crisis standards of care for use in disaster situations: A letter report.* Washington, DC: The National Academies Press.

Levin, D., R. O. Cadigan, P. D. Biddinger, S. Condon, and H. K. Koh. 2009. Altered standards of care during an influenza pandemic: Identifying ethical, legal, and practical principles to guide decision making. *Disaster Med Public Health Prep.* http://www.dmphp.org/ (accessed September 14, 2009).

Lieberman, D., Nachshon, L., Miloslavsky, O., Dvorkin, V., Shimoni, A., and D. Lieberman. 2009. How do older ventilated patients fare? A survival/functional analysis of 641 ventilations. *J Crit Care* 24(3):340–346.

Matzo, M. L. 2004. Palliative care: Prognostication and the chronically ill: Methods you need to know as chronic disease progresses in older adults. *Am J Nurs* 104(9):40–49; quiz 50.

Minnesota Department of Health. 2008. *Minnesota healthcare system preparedness program standards of care for scarce resources.* http://www.health.state.mn.us/oep/healthcare/standards.pdf (accessed September 8, 2009).

Mitchell, S. L., D. K. Kiely, M. B. Hamel, P. S. Park, J. N. Morris, and B. E. Fries. 2004. Estimating prognosis for nursing home residents with advanced dementia. *JAMA* 291(22):2734–2740.

New Jersey Hospital Association. 2008. *Planning today for a pandemic tomorrow: Video vignettes.* http://www.njha.com/paninf/index.aspx (accessed September 8, 2009).

O'Laughlin, D. T., and J. L. Hick. 2008. Ethical issues in resource triage. *Respir Care* 53(2):190–197; discussion 197–200.

Ontario Ministry of Health and Long-term Care. 2008. *Ontario health plan for an influenza pandemic.* http://www.health.gov.on.ca/english/providers/program/emu/pan_flu/pan_flu_plan.html#section (accessed September 8, 2009).

Phillips, S., and A. Knebel, eds. 2007. *Mass medical care with scarce resources: A community planning guide.* AHRQ Publication No. 07-0001. Rockville, MD: AHRQ.

Powell, T., K. C. Christ, and G. S. Birkhead. 2008. Allocation of ventilators in a public health disaster. *Disaster Med Public Health Prep* 2(1):20–26.

PricewaterhouseCoopers. 2007. *Closing the seams: Developing an integrated approach to health system disaster preparedness.* http://www.pwc.com/us/en/healthcare/publications/closing-the-seams.jhtml (accessed November 2, 2009).

The Commonwealth of Massachusetts Department of Public Health. 2007 (unpublished). *Guidelines for the development of altered standards of care for influenza pandemic.*

The Utah Hospitals and Health Systems Association. 2009. *Utah pandemic influenza hospital and ICU triage guidelines. Version 1.* http://www.pandemicflu.utah.gov/plan/med_triage011009.pdf (accessed September 8, 2009).

VHA (Veterans Health Administration). 2008a (unpublished). *Tertiary triage protocol for allocation of scarce life-saving resources in VHA during an influenza pandemic.*

VHA. 2008b. *VA staff discussion forums on ethics issues in pandemic influenza preparedness.* http://www.ethics.va.gov/activities/pandemic_influenza_preparedness.asp (accessed September 30, 2009).

VHA. 2009a (unpublished). *Draft guidance: Meeting the challenge of pandemic influenza: Ethical guidance for VHA leaders and clinicians.*

VHA. 2009b. *IntegratedEthics Program.* http://www.ethics.va.gov/integrated/ethics/index.asp (accessed September 30, 2009).

Virginia Department of Health. 2008. *Virginia Hospital and Healthcare Association Altered Standards of Care Workgroup: Critical resource shortages: A planning guide.* http://www.troutmansanders.com/files/upload/Critical%20Resource%20Shortages-A%20Planning%20Guide.pdf (accessed September 8, 2009).

Walter, L. C., R. J. Brand, S. R. Counsell, R. M. Palmer, C. S. Landefeld, R. H. Fortinsky, and K. E. Covinsky. 2001. Development and validation of a prognostic index for 1-year mortality in older adults after hospitalization. *JAMA* 285(23):2987–2994.

Washington State Department of Health's Altered Standards of Care Workgroup. 2008 (unpublished). *Report and recommendations to the Department of Health Secretary on establishing altered standards of care during an influenza pandemic.*

Wynia, M. 2009. *IOM Committee on Guidance for Establishing Standards of Care for Use in Disaster Situations.* Paper presented at IOM Committee on Guidance for Establishing Standards of Care for Use in Disaster Situations, September 2, Washington, DC.

# B

# Summary of
## *Guidance for Establishing Crisis Standards of Care for Use in Disaster Situations: A Letter Report*

At the request of the Office of the Assistant Secretary for Preparedness and Response in the Department of Health and Human Services, the Institute of Medicine convened the Committee on Guidance for Establishing Standards of Care for Use in Disaster Situations to develop guidance that state and local public health officials can use to establish and implement standards of care that should apply in disaster situations—both naturally occurring and manmade—under scarce resource conditions. Specifically, the committee was asked to identify and describe the key elements that should be included in crisis standards of care protocols, to identify potential indicators and triggers, and to develop a template matrix that can be used by state and local public health officials as a framework for developing specific guidance for healthcare provider communities to develop and implement crisis standards of care. This appendix provides a summary of the committee's recommendations, findings, and practical guidance. A complete copy of the report is available through www.iom.edu/disasterstandards.

Based on a review of the currently available state standards of care protocols, published literature, and testimony provided at its workshop, the committee concluded that there is an urgent and clear need for a single national set of guidance for states with crisis standards of care that can be generalized to all crisis events and is not specific to a certain event. However, the committee recognizes that within such a single general framework, individual disaster scenarios may require specific considerations, such as differences between no-notice events and slow-onset events, while the key elements and components remain the same.

For the purpose of developing recommendations for situations in which healthcare resources are overwhelmed, the committee defined the level of health and medical care capable of being delivered during a catastrophic event as "crisis standards of care."

> *"Crisis standards of care" is defined as a substantial change in usual healthcare operations and the level of care it is possible to deliver, which is made necessary by a pervasive (e.g., pandemic influenza) or catastrophic (e.g., earthquake, hurricane) disaster. This change in the level of care delivered is justified by specific circumstances and is formally declared by a state government, in recognition that crisis operations will be in effect for a sustained period. The formal declaration that crisis standards of care are in operation enables specific legal/regulatory powers and protections for healthcare providers in the necessary tasks of allocating and using scarce medical resources and implementing alternate care facility operations.*

The committee emphasized that, in an important ethical sense, entering a crisis standard of care mode is not optional—it is a forced choice, based on the emerging situation. Under such circumstances, failing to make substantive adjustments to care operations—that is, not to adopt crisis standards of care—is very likely to result in greater death, injury, or illness.


## THE VISION

In order to ensure that patients receive the best possible care in a catastrophic event, the nation needs a robust system to guide the public, healthcare professionals and institutions, and governmental entities at all levels. To achieve such a system of just care, the committee set forth the following vision for crisis standards of care:

- *Fairness*—standards that are, to the highest degree possible, recognized as fair by all those affected by them (including the members of affected communities, practitioners, and provider organizations); evidence based; and responsive to specific needs of individuals and the population focused on a duty of compassion and care, a duty to steward resources, and a goal of maintaining the trust of patients and the community

- *Equitable processes*—processes and procedures for ensuring that decisions and implementation of standards are made equitably
  - o Transparency—in design and decision making
  - o Consistency—in application across populations and among individuals regardless of their human condition (e.g., race, age, disability, ethnicity, ability to pay, socioeconomic status, preexisting health conditions, social worth, perceived obstacles to treatment, past use of resources)
  - o Proportionality—public and individual requirements must be commensurate with the scale of the emergency and degree of scarce resources
  - o Accountability—of individuals deciding and implementing standards, and of governments for ensuring appropriate protections and just allocation of available resources
- *Community and provider engagement, education, and communication*—active collaboration with the public and stakeholders for their input is essential through formalized processes
- *The rule of law*
  - o Authority—to empower necessary and appropriate actions and interventions in response to emergencies
  - o Environment—to facilitate implementation through laws that support standards and create appropriate incentives

## DEVELOPING CRISIS STANDARDS OF CARE PROTOCOLS

Throughout the report, the committee emphasized the need for states to develop and implement consistent crisis standards of care protocols both within the state and through work with neighboring states, in collaboration with their partners in the public and private sectors. The committee's intent was to provide a framework that allows consistency in establishing the key components required of any effort focused on crisis standards of care in a disaster situation. It also hoped that by suggesting a uniform approach, consistency will develop across geographic and political boundaries so that the guidance will be useful in contributing to a single, national framework for responding to crises in a fair, equitable, and transparent manner.

**Recommendation 1: <u>Develop Consistent State Crisis Standards of Care Protocols with Five Key Elements</u>** **State departments of health, and other relevant state agencies, in partnership with localities should develop crisis standards of care protocols that include the key elements—and associated components—detailed in this report:**

- **A strong ethical grounding;**
- **Integrated and ongoing community and provider engagement, education, and communication;**
- **Assurances regarding legal authority and environment;**
- **Clear indicators, triggers, and lines of responsibility; and**
- **Evidence-based clinical processes and operations.**

The report also contains guidance to assist state public health authorities in developing these crisis standards of care. This guidance includes criteria for determining when crisis standards of care should be implemented, key elements that should be included in the crisis standards of care protocols, and criteria for determining when these standards of care should be implemented. The five key elements that should be included in crisis standards of care protocols, along with associated components, are summarized in Table B-1.

**TABLE B-1** Five Key Elements of Crisis Standards of Care Protocols and Associated Components

| Key Elements of Crisis Standards of Care Protocols | Components |
|---|---|
| Ethical considerations | <ul><li>Fairness</li><li>Duty to care</li><li>Duty to steward resources</li><li>Transparency</li><li>Consistency</li><li>Proportionality</li><li>Accountability</li></ul> |
| Community and provider engagement, education, and communication | <ul><li>Community stakeholder identification with delineation of roles and involvement with attention to vulnerable populations</li><li>Community trust and assurance of fairness and transparency in processes developed</li></ul> |

| Key Elements of Crisis Standards of Care Protocols | Components |
|---|---|
| | • Community cultural values and boundaries<br>• Continuum of community education and trust building<br>• Crisis risk communication strategies and situational awareness<br>• Continuum of resilience building and mental health triage<br>• Palliative care education for stakeholders |
| Legal authority and environment | • Medical and legal standards of care<br>• Scope of practice for healthcare professionals<br>• Mutual aid agreements to facilitate resource allocation<br>• Federal, state, and local declarations of:<br>   ○ Emergency<br>   ○ Disaster<br>   ○ Public health emergency<br>• Special emergency protections (e.g., PREP Act, Section 1135 waivers of sanctions under EMTALA and HIPAA Privacy Rule)<br>• Licensing and credentialing<br>• Medical malpractice<br>• Liability risks (civil, criminal, Constitutional)<br>• Statutory, regulatory, and common-law liability protections |
| Indicators and triggers | Indicators for assessment and potential management<br>• Situational awareness (local/regional, state, national)<br>• Event specific<br>   ○ Illness and injury—incidence and severity<br>   ○ Disruption of social and community functioning<br>   ○ Resource availability<br><br>Triggers for action<br>• Critical infrastructure disruption<br>• Failure of "contingency" surge capacity (resource-sparing strategies overwhelmed)<br>   ○ Human resource/staffing availability<br>   ○ Material resource availability<br>   ○ Patient care space availability |

| Key Elements of Crisis Standards of Care Protocols | Components |
|---|---|
| Clinical process and operations | Local/regional and state government processes to include: <br> • State-level "disaster medical advisory committee" and local "clinical care committees" and "triage teams" <br> • Resource-sparing strategies <br> • Incident management (NIMS/HICS) principles <br> • Intrastate and interstate regional consistencies in the application of crisis standards of care <br> • Coordination of resource management <br> • Specific attention to vulnerable populations and those with medical special needs <br> • Communications strategies <br> • Coordination extends through all elements of the health system, including public health, emergency medical services, long-term care, primary care, and home care <br><br> Clinical operations based on crisis surge response plan: <br> • Decision support tool to triage life-sustaining interventions <br> • Palliative care principles <br> • Mental health needs and promotion of resilience |

The letter report states that "state authorities have the political and constitutional mandate to prepare for and coordinate the response to disaster situations throughout their state jurisdictions" and outlines a process by which states should begin to develop crisis standards of care protocols. These steps include the following:

1. Outline Ethical Considerations: Convene a "Guideline Development Working Group" of appropriate stakeholders to establish ethical principles that will serve as the basis for the crisis standards of care.

2. Review Legal Authority for Implementation of Crisis Standards of Care: Review existing legal authority for the implementation of crisis standards of care and address legal issues related to the successful implementation of these standards, such as liability

protections or temporary changes in licensure or certification status or scope of practice.

3. Develop Guidance for Provision of Medical Care Under State Crisis Standards of Care: Establish an "Advisory Committee" that will find a comprehensive set of materials to inform its deliberations in the "Indicators and Triggers" and "Clinical Process and Operations" sections of the report.

4. Conduct a Public Stakeholder Engagement Process: Although representatives of various healthcare and other interested professional groups and the public have been involved in drafting the ethical principles and crisis standards of care, a robust engagement process is also necessary to provide an opportunity for review and comment by the provider and public community at large. Particular attention should be paid to conduct outreach to and gather input from vulnerable populations, including those with medical special needs.

5. Establish a Medical Disaster Advisory Committee: During a disaster, this committee will provide ongoing advice to the state authority regarding changes to the situation and potential corresponding changes in the implementation of crisis standards of care.

## ETHICAL FRAMEWORK

An ethical framework serves as the bedrock for public policy and cannot be added as an afterthought. Hence, ethical principles underlie the committee's vision for crisis planning, outlined above. In addition, ethically and clinically sound planning will aim to secure fair and equitable resources and protections for vulnerable groups. The committee concluded that core ethical precepts in medicine permit some actions during crisis situations that would not be acceptable under ordinary circumstances, such as implementing resource allocation protocols that could preclude the use of certain resources on some patients when others would derive greater benefit from them. But even here, it is the situation that changes during disasters, not ethical standards per se. The context of a disaster may make certain resources unavailable for some or even all patients, but it does not provide license to act without regard to professional or legal standards. Healthcare professionals are obligated always to provide the best care they reasonably can to each patient in their care, including during crises. When resource scarcity reaches catastrophic levels, clinicians are ethically justified—and indeed are ethically obligated—to use the available resources to sustain life and well-being to the greatest extent possible. As a result, the committee concluded that ethics permits clinicians to allocate scarce resources so as to provide necessary and available treatments preferentially to those patients most likely to benefit when operating under crisis standards of care. However, operating under crisis standards of care does not permit clinicians to ignore professional norms nor to act without ethical standards or accountability.

> **Recommendation: Adhere to Ethical Norms During Crisis Standards of Care**
> **When crisis standards of care prevail, as when ordinary standards are in effect, healthcare practitioners must adhere to ethical norms. Conditions of overwhelming scarcity limit autonomous choices for both patients and practitioners regarding the allocation of scarce healthcare resources, but do not permit actions that violate ethical norms.**

## COMMUNITY AND PROVIDER ENGAGEMENT, EDUCATION, AND COMMUNICATION

The committee strongly recommended extensive engagement with community and provider stakeholders. Such public engagement is necessary not only to ensure the legitimacy of the process and standards, but more importantly to achieve the best possible result. The letter report discusses considerations for engaging with community and provider stakeholders prior to the event, during the event, and after the event. The report also notes that although there are likely to be substantive population-level mental health risks from a mass casualty public health emergency that requires crisis standards of care, there is also an opportunity to promote resilience at the individual and population levels to mitigate these risks. Thus it is important to develop a national platform to support resilience that can customized by communities at the local level. The report also emphasizes that building trust is particularly important in more vulnerable populations, including those with preexisting health inequities and those with unique needs related to race, ethnicity, culture, immigration, limited English proficiency, and lower socioeconomic status.

**Recommendation: <u>Seek Community and Provider Engagement</u>**
**State, local, and tribal governments should partner with and work to ensure strong public engagement of community and provider stakeholders, with particular attention given to the needs of vulnerable populations and those with medical special needs, in:**

- **Developing and refining crisis standards of care protocols and implementation guidance;**
- **Creating and disseminating educational tools and messages to both the public and health professionals;**
- **Developing and implementing crisis communication strategies;**
- **Developing and implementing community resilience strategies; and**
- **Learning from and improving crisis standards of care response situations.**

## LEGAL ISSUES IN EMERGENCIES

The letter report also addressed issues related to the implementation of crisis standards of care, including legal considerations. Questions of legal empowerment of various actions to protect individual and communal health are pervasive and complicated by interjurisdictional inconsistencies. The law should clarify prevailing standards of care and create incentives for actors to respond to protect the public's health and respect individual rights.

**Recommendation: <u>Provide Necessary Legal Protections for Healthcare Practitioners and Institutions Implementing Crisis Standards of Care</u>**
**In disaster situations, tribal or state governments should authorize appropriate agencies to institute crisis standards of care in affected areas, adjust scopes of**

practice for licensed or certified healthcare practitioners, and alter licensure and credentialing practices as
needed in declared emergencies to create incentives to
provide care needed for the health of individuals and
the public.

## OPERATIONAL IMPLEMENTATION OF
## CRISIS STANDARDS OF CARE

### Clinical Care in Disasters

An important consideration regarding the framework for the implementation of crisis standards of care in a disaster includes the recognition
that it will never be an "all or none" situation. Disasters will have vary-
ing impacts on communities, based on many different variables that
might affect the delivery of health care during such events. Response to a
surge in demand for healthcare services will likely fall along a continuum ranging from "conventional" to "contingency" and "crisis" surge
responses (Figure B-1; Hick et al., 2009). Conventional patient care uses
usual resources to deliver health and medical care that conforms to the
expected standards of care of the community. The delivery of care in the
setting of contingency surge response seeks to provide patient care that
remains *functionally equivalent* to conventional care. Contingency care
adapts available patient care spaces, staff, and supplies as part of the response to a surge in demand for services. Although this may introduce
minor risk to the patient compared to usual care (e.g., substituting less
familiar medications for those in short supply, thereby potentially leading
to medication dosage error), the overall delivery of care remains mostly
consistent with community standards. Crisis care, however, occurs under
conditions in which usual safeguards are no longer possible. Crisis care
is provided when available resources are insufficient to meet usual care
standards, thus providing a transition point to implementing *crisis standards of care.*

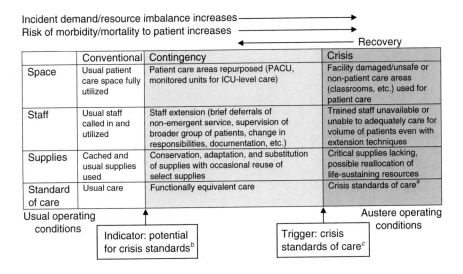

FIGURE B-1 Continuum of incident care and implications for standards of care.

NOTE: Post-anesthesia care unit (PACU); intensive care unit (ICU).

[a]Unless temporary, requires state empowerment, clinical guidance, and protection for triage decisions and authorization for alternate care sites/techniques. Once situational awareness achieved, triage decisions should be as systematic and integrated into institutional process, review, and documentation as possible.

[b]Institutions consider impact on the community of resource use (consider "greatest good" versus individual patient needs—e.g., conserve resources when possible), but patient-centered decision making is still the focus.

[c]Institutions (and providers) must make triage decisions balancing the availability of resources to others and the individual patient's needs—shift to community-centered decision making.

SOURCES: Adapted from Hick et al. (2009); Wynia (2009).

The goal for the health system is to increase the ability to stay in conventional and contingency categories through preparedness and anticipation of resource needs prior to serious shortages, and to return as quickly as possible from crisis back across the continuum to conventional care (Tables B-2 and B-3).

**TABLE B-2** Sample Strategies to Address Resource Shortages

|            | Conventional Capacity | Contingency Capacity | Crisis Capacity |
|------------|----------------------|----------------------|-----------------|
| Prepare    | Stockpile supplies used | | |
| Substitute | Equivalent medications used (narcotic substitution) | | |
| Conserve   | Oxygen flow rates titrated to minimum required, discontinued for saturations > 95% | Oxygen only for saturations < 90% | Oxygen only for respiratory failure |
| Adapt      | | Anesthesia machine for mechanical ventilation | Bag valve manual ventilation |
| Reuse      | Reuse cervical collars after surface disinfection | Reuse nasogastric tubes and ventilator circuits after appropriate disinfection | Reuse invasive lines after appropriate sterilization |
| Reallocate | | Reallocate oxygen saturation monitors, cardiac monitors, only to those with critical illness | Reallocate ventilators to those with the best chance of a good outcome |

SOURCE: Adapted from Hick et al. (2009).

**TABLE B-3** Sample Strategies for Emergency Medical Services (EMS) Agencies to Address Resource Shortages

| EMS Agency Resources | Contingency Changes | Crisis: Implement Contingency Changes Plus |
|----------------------|---------------------|--------------------------------------------|
| Dispatch | Assign single agency responses, use medical priority dispatch to decline services to select calls | Assign EMS only to life-threatening calls by predetermined criteria, no response to cardiopulmonary resuscitation-in-progress calls, questions may be altered to receive limited critical information from caller |
| Staffing | Adjust shift length and staffing patterns | One medical provider per unit plus driver |
| Response | "Batch" calls (multiple patients transported), closest hospital destination | No resuscitation on cardiac arrest calls, decline service to noncritical, nonvulnerable patients and to critical patients with little to no chance of survival |

## Disaster Mental Health Crisis Standards of Care

In major disaster and emergencies, there will also be a surge of psychological casualties among those directly affected, including responders, healthcare practitioners, and members of the population who have not experienced direct impact. Mass psychological casualties and morbidity will occur in those who experience an aggravation of a prior or concurrent mental health condition. New substantial burdens of clinical disorders, including posttraumatic stress disorder, depression, and substance abuse may also arise among those with no prior history. Even in those with no formal disorder, there may be significant distress at a population level, resulting in unparalleled demands on the mental health system. Therefore, it is necessary to use a mass casualty disaster mental health concept of operations in order to enable a crisis standard of disaster mental health care through the use of currently available, evidence-based mental health rapid triage and incident management systems. Additional details can be found in the complete letter report.

## Palliative Care Planning for Crisis Standards of Care

Providing a treatment category of "palliative care" for those not likely to survive will be an important service option for responders and triage officers. Acknowledging that a patient is not likely to survive typically leads to discussions regarding the goals of care, appropriateness of interventions, and efforts to help the patient and family begin to say good-bye (Matzo, 2004). Prognostication, aided by a risk index or scale, enables healthcare practitioners to plan clinical strategies during a crisis situation. These tools may be helpful in determining whether a patient's illness has reached a terminal phase (Box B-1) (Matzo, 2004).

---

**BOX B-1**
**Palliative Care Triage Tools**

**Flacker Mortality Score:** Flacker and Kiely developed a model for identifying factors associated with one-year mortality (the probability of death within the next year) by conducting a retrospective cohort study using Minimum Data Set (MDS) information from residents in a 725-bed, long-term care facility (Flacker and Kiely, 1998). The Flacker Mortality Score instrument is the risk-assessment scale developed from those findings. It is used in conjunction with MDS data collected using the standard Resident

Assessment Instrument and is applicable to *elders living in long-term care facilities* (Matzo, 2004; CMS, 2002).

**Risk Index for Older Adults:** The Risk Index for Older Adults establishes point scores for several risk factors associated with death within one year of hospital discharge and allows a clinician to evaluate a patient's risk of death accordingly. The point system is based on a study of 2,922 patients discharged from an acute care hospital (Walter et al., 2001). The researchers concluded that, in predicting one-year mortality, this index performed better than other prognostic scales that focus only on coexisting illnesses or physiologic measures. It takes into consideration a cancer diagnosis and is *applicable to hospitalized elders* (Matzo, 2004).

**Mortality Risk Index:** A recent study by Mitchell and colleagues identified factors associated with the 6-month mortality of nursing home residents diagnosed with advanced dementia (Mitchell et al., 2004). The retrospective study of MDS data from 11,430 patients with advanced dementia admitted to nursing homes in New York and Michigan generated risk scores based on 12 MDS variables. The researchers concluded that these risk scores provided more accurate estimates of 6-month mortality than those derived from existing prognostic guidelines (Matzo, 2004).

## Crisis Standards of Care Indicators

Resources that are likely to be scarce in a crisis care environment and may justify specific planning and tracking include the following:

- Ventilators and components
- Oxygen and oxygen delivery devices
- Vascular access devices
- Intensive care unit (ICU) beds
- Healthcare providers, particularly critical care, burn, and surgical/anesthesia staff (nurses and physicians) and respiratory therapists
- Hospitals (due to infrastructure damage or compromise)
- Specialty medications or intravenous fluids (sedatives/analgesics, specific antibiotics, antivirals, etc.)
- Vasopressors/inotropes
- Medical transportation

The committee discussed the need to consider both indicators and triggers:

Indicator—measurement or predictor that is used to recognize capacity and capability problems within the healthcare system, suggesting that crisis standards of care may become necessary and requiring further analysis or system actions to prevent overload (Table B-4).

Trigger—evidence of use of crisis standard of care practices that require an institutional, and often regional, response to ameliorate the situation (Table B-5).

**TABLE B-4** Possible Indicators for Crisis Capacity[a]

| Indicators | Institution/ Agency | Region | State |
|---|---|---|---|
| Situational awareness indicators | | | |
| Overall hospital bed availability | < 5% available or no available beds for >12 hours | < 5% | < 5% |
| Intensive care unit bed availability | None available | < 5% regional beds available | < 5% state beds available |
| Ventilators | < 5% available | < 5% available | < 5% available |
| Divert status | On divert > 12 hours | > 50% EDs on divert | > 50% EDs on divert |
| Emergency medical services call volume | 2 times usual | | |
| Syndromic predictions | Will exceed capacity | Will exceed capacity | Will exceed capacity |
| Emergency department (ED) wait time | > 12 hours | | |
| Event-specific indicators | | | |
| Illness/injury incidence and severity | | | |
| Disaster declaration | | > 1 area hospital | > 2 major hospitals |

| Indicators | Institution/ Agency | Region | State |
|---|---|---|---|
| Contingency care being provided and unable to rapidly address shortfall | Any hospital reporting | Any hospital reporting | Any hospital reporting |
| Resource-specific shortage (e.g., antibiotic, immunoglobulin, oxygen, vaccine) | Notification by supplier | Notification by hospitals | Notification by hospitals/ suppliers |
| Outpatient care | Marked increase in appointment demand or unable to reach clinic due to call volume | | |
| Staff illness rate | > 10% | > 10% | > 10% |
| School Absenteeism | Not applicable | > 20% | > 20% |
| Disruption of facility or community infrastructure and function | Utility or system failure | > 1 hospital affected | > 5 hospitals affected or critical access hospital affected |

[a]The indicators in this table should be developed in relation to usual resources in the area and usage patterns—*numbers are examples only.*


**TABLE B-5** Possible Triggers for Adjusting Standards of Care

| Category | Trigger |
|---|---|
| Space/structure | Non-patient care locations used for patient care (e.g., cot-based care, care in lobby areas) or specific space resources overwhelmed (operating rooms) and delay presents a significant risk of morbidity or mortality; or disrupted or unsafe facility infrastructure (damage, systems failure) |
| Staff | Specialty staff unavailable in timely manner to provide or adequately supervise care (pediatric, burn, surgery, critical care) even after callback procedures have been implemented |
| Supply | Supplies absent or unable to substitute, leading to risk to patient of morbidity (including untreated pain) or mortality (e.g., absence of available ventilators, lack of specific antibiotics) |

## Crisis Standards of Care Implementation Criteria

Prior to implementation of formal resource triage, the following conditions must be met or in process (Devereaux et al., 2008):

- Identification of critically limited resources and infrastructure
- Surge capacity fully employed within healthcare facility
- Maximal attempts at conservation, reuse, adaptation, and substitution performed
- Regional, state, and federal resource allocation insufficient to meet demand
- Patient transfer or resource importation not possible or will occur too late to consider bridging therapies
- Request for necessary resources made to local and regional health officials
- Declared state of emergency (or in process)

## Crisis Standards of Care Triage

Triage occurs routinely in medicine, when resources are not evenly distributed or temporarily overwhelmed. These decisions are generally ad hoc, based on provider expertise, and have minimal effects on patient outcome. Thus standards of care are routinely adjusted to resources available to the provider without requiring a formal process or declarations. However, the situation in disasters is more complex, as services may not be available due to demand, with severe consequences to the patient who does not receive these resources. Reactive triage involves the ad hoc decisions made by clinical or administrative personnel to an exigent circumstance to allocate available resources in the face of an unanticipated shortfall. These decisions must be accountable to general principles of ethical resource allocation, but do not follow a structured, systematic process. Situational awareness is not available. Proactive triage involves systematic decisions made by clinical or administrative personnel to a situation requiring resource triage where situational awareness is available and the decision making is accountable to the incident management process. Additional details about reactive and proactive triage are available in the letter report.

## Prerequisite Command, Control, and Coordination Elements

The implementation of crisis standards of care and fair and equitable resource allocation requires attention to the core elements of incident management, including situational awareness, incident command, and adequate communication and coordination infrastructure and policies. Without this foundation, medical care will be inconsistent, and resources will not be optimally used (Hick et al., 2009). All healthcare systems must also understand how their incident management system interacts with that of jurisdictional emergency management and any coalition hospital response partners, including the process for obtaining assistance during an emergency (Figure B-2).

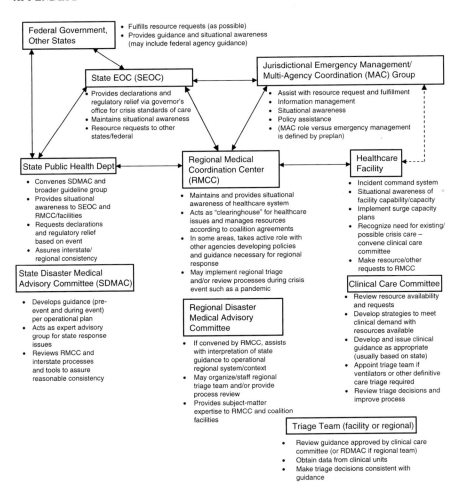

**FIGURE B-2** Overview of relationships among agencies, committees, and groups.
NOTE: Depending on the organization of the state, the functional layout, details, and relationships among the units might vary.

## Crisis Standards of Care Operations

When crisis care becomes necessary, a threshold has been crossed requiring that the affected institution(s) either quickly address the situation internally, or, more likely, appeal to partner facilities and agencies for assistance in either transferring patients to facilities with resources or bringing needed resources to the facility. If these strategies cannot be carried out, or if partner facilities are in the same situation (e.g., a pandemic influenza scenario), then systematic implementation of crisis standards of care at the state level may become necessary in order to codify and provide guidance for triage of life-sustaining interventions as well as to authorize care provided in non-traditional locations (alternate care facilities).

The state has an obligation to ensure consistency of medical care to the highest degree possible when crisis care is being provided. Usual coordination and resource requests outlined above are used to minimize healthcare service disruption and/or to provide the most consistent level of care across the affected area and the state as a whole. When prolonged or widespread crisis care is necessary, the state should issue a declaration or invoke emergency powers empowering and protecting providers and agencies to take necessary actions to provide medical care *and* should accompany these declarations with clinical guidance, developed by the State Disaster Medical Advisory Committee, to provide a consistent basis for life-sustaining resource allocation decisions. The state, through its emergency powers, resource allocation, and provision of clinical guidance, attempts to "level the playing field" at the state level, as well as provide legal protections for providers making difficult triage decisions and provide relief from usual regulations that might impede coping strategies such as alternate care facilities.

Some hospital coalitions cover large metropolitan areas and thus the Regional Medical Coordination Center (RMCC) acts as liaison between the state and its constituents. The RMCC may be an agency, such as public health, or a hospital or other facility designated by the system. The RMCC attempts to ensure regional medical care consistency and may do so by acting as a resource "clearinghouse" between the healthcare facilities and emergency management and coordinating policy and information to meet regional needs. This may involve a Regional Disaster Medical Advisory Committee or at least a medical advisor or coordinator with access to technical experts in the area, particularly in large metropolitan areas because the specific needs of the area may not be well addressed by state guidance. However, the regional guidance cannot be *inconsistent* with that of the state.

Individual hospitals and healthcare facilities should work through tactical mutual aid agreements with other local facilities and at the regional level to ameliorate conditions that might force crisis standards of care. When these strategies have been exhausted, healthcare facilities, working through local public health authorities, should request a state emergency declaration recognizing that crisis conditions are at hand, that a change in acceptable standards of care are required, and that crisis standards of care must be initiated.

The individual healthcare institution surge capacity plan should incorporate the use of a "clinical care committee" that is composed of clinical and administrative leaders who can focus a hospital or hospital system approach to the allocation of scarce, life-saving resources (Phillips and Knebel, 2007; Hick and O'Laughlin, 2006; O'Laughlin and Hick, 2008). A clinical care committee is activated by the facility incident commander when the facility is practicing contingency or crisis care due to factors that are not readily reversible. This committee is responsible for making prioritization decisions about the use of resources at the relevant healthcare institution (e.g., hospital, primary care, emergency medical services agency, and others). A sample institutional process is included in the letter report.

## Decision Tools and Resource Use Guidance

Although the most examined decision tools revolve around mechanical ventilation, guidance is also available for other core medical care components (medications, oxygen, etc.) and limited guidance is available for specific other resources, including blood products, elective surgery triage, trauma care, radiation, burn care, and cancer (Box B-2, Figure B-3). See the letter report for additional details.

**BOX B-2**
**Exclusion Criteria Prompting Possible Reallocation of Life-Saving Interventions**

**Sequential Organ Failure Assessment (SOFA) score criteria:** patients excluded from critical care if risk of hospital mortality > 80%
  A.  SOFA > 15
  B.  SOFA > 5 for >5 d, and with flat or rising trend
  C.  > 6 organ failures

**Severe, chronic disease with a short life expectancy**
  A.  Severe trauma
  B.  Severe burns on patient with any two of the following:
    i.   Age > 60 yr
    ii.  > 40% of total body surface area affected
    iii. Inhalational injury
  C.  Cardiac arrest
    i.   Unwitnessed cardiac arrest
    ii.  Witnessed cardiac arrest, not responsive to electrical therapy (defibrillation or pacing)
    iii. Recurrent cardiac arrest
  D.  Severe baseline cognitive impairment
  E.  Advanced untreatable neuromuscular disease
  F.  Metastatic malignant disease
  G.  Advanced and irreversible neurologic event or condition
  H.  End-stage organ failure (for details see Devereaux et al., 2008)
  I.  Age > 85 yr (see Lieberman et al., 2009)
  J.  Elective palliative surgery

SOURCE: Adapted from Devereaux et al. (2008).

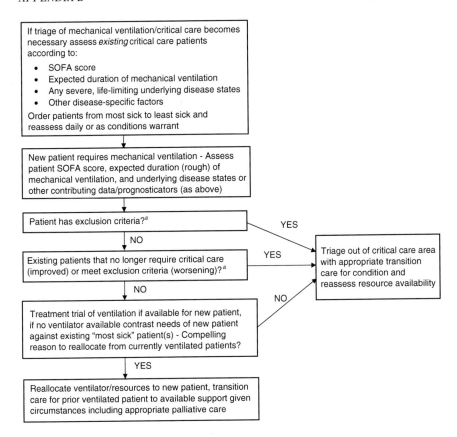

**FIGURE B-3** Triage algorithm process.
[a]Example exclusion criteria include severe, irreversible organ failure (congestive heart failure, liver, etc.), severe neurologic compromise, extremely high or not improving SOFA scores, etc.
SOURCE: Adapted from Devereaux et al. (2008).

Finally, throughout the letter report, the committee emphasized the importance of consistent implementation of crisis standards of care in a disaster situation within and among states.

> **Recommendation: <u>Ensure Consistency in Crisis Standards of Care Implementation</u>**
> **State departments of health, and other relevant state agencies, in partnership with localities should ensure consistent implementation of crisis standards of care**

in response to a disaster event. These efforts should include:

- Using "clinical care committees," "triage teams," and a state-level "disaster medical advisory committee" that will evaluate evidence-based, peer-reviewed critical care and other decision tools and recommend and implement decision-making algorithms to be used when specific life-sustaining resources become scarce;
- Providing palliative care services for all patients, including the provision of comfort, compassion, and maintenance of dignity;
- Mobilizing mental health resources to help communities—and providers themselves—to manage the effects of crisis standards of care by following a concept of operations developed for disasters;
- Developing specific response measures for vulnerable populations and those with medical special needs, including pediatrics, geriatrics, and persons with disabilities; and
- Implementing robust situational awareness capabilities to allow for real-time information sharing across affected communities and with the "disaster medical advisory committee."

Recommendation: Ensure Intrastate and Interstate Consistency Among Neighboring Jurisdictions
States, in partnership with the federal government, tribes, and localities, should initiate communications and develop processes to ensure intrastate and interstate consistency in the implementation of crisis standards of care. Specific efforts are needed to ensure that the Department of Defense, Veterans Health Administration, and Indian Health Service medical facilities are integrated into planning and response efforts.

## CONCLUSION

Crisis standards of care, as described in the report, will be required when the intent and ability to provide usual care is simply no longer possible due to the circumstances. As acknowledged by the committee, some governments have made great strides in determining how to approach resource scarcity, but much work remains to be done.

Indeed, the committee highlighted a number of areas worthy of further discussion, evaluation, and study. Some of these issues constitute real or perceived barriers that will make the implementation and operationalization of crisis standards of care difficult to achieve. Some simply reflect the fact that the study of this area of disaster medicine remains an evolving pursuit requiring multidisciplinary participation. Nonetheless, the discussion around this topic has matured tremendously in the past few years. Despite the gaps that remain, the committee was greatly encouraged by the search for solutions taking place.

In studying this issue, the committee's intent was to provide a framework that allows consistency in describing the key components required by any effort focused on standards of care in a disaster. It also intended that, by suggesting such uniformity, consistency will develop across jurisdictions, regions, and states so that this guidance will be useful in contributing to a uniform national framework for responding to crisis in a fair, equitable, and transparent manner.

# C

# Workshop Agendas[1]

Irvine Workshop
March 12, 2009
The Beckman Center
Irvine, CA


Orlando Workshop
April 14, 2009
Disney's Coronado Springs Resort
Lake Buena Vista, FL


New York Workshop
April 27, 2009
Albert Einstein College of Medicine
Bronx, NY


Chicago Workshop
May 8, 2009
American Medical Association
Chicago, IL

---

[1]To save space, the individual agendas from each regional meeting have been compiled into a single document. Under each session speakers have been identified based on each meeting location at which they participated: Irvine, Orlando, New York, and/or Chicago.

## Workshop Objectives:

- Illuminate the progress and successes of efforts underway to establish local, state, and regional standards of care protocols.
  - What have been some of the barriers in establishing protocols?
  - What solutions have been developed to operationalize standards of care protocols?
- Improve regional efforts by facilitating a dialogue and coordination among neighboring jurisdictions.
- Discuss the roles and responsibilities of each stakeholder community in the development and implementation of standards of care protocols, including officials from state and local health departments and providers.
- Examine what resources, guidelines, and expertise have been used to establish standards of care protocols, including legal and ethical expertise that has been used to establish standards of care protocols.
- Identify and discuss resource requirements that will be necessary from federal, state, and regional authorities to advance and accelerate the establishment of standards of care protocols.


## Welcoming Remarks

*New York*
DEAN ALLEN SPIEGEL, Albert Einstein College of Medicine of Yeshiva University

*Chicago*
JAMES J. JAMES, American Medical Association


## Welcome, Introductions, and Workshop Objectives

*Irvine, Orlando, New York, Chicago*
SALLY PHILLIPS, Agency for Healthcare Research and Quality, *Workshop Chair*

## SESSION I: OVERVIEW AND CURRENT NATIONAL EFFORTS

<u>Session Objective:</u> Provide an overview of current efforts under way nationally to assist state and local leaders in establishing standards of care protocols.

### Standards of Care During a Mass Casualty Event—Federal Guidance

*Irvine, Orlando, New York, Chicago*
    SALLY PHILLIPS, Agency for Healthcare Research and Quality,
    *Workshop Chair*

### Surge Capacity Continuum: Conventional, Contingency, and Crisis

*Irvine, Chicago*
    JOHN HICK, Hennepin County Medical Center, MN

*Orlando, New York*
    DAN HANFLING, Inova Health System

### Altered Standards of Care Continuum: Conventional, Contingency, and Crisis

*Irvine, Orlando, New York, Chicago*
    DAN HANFLING, Inova Health System

### Framing Legal and Ethical Considerations

*Irvine*
    CHERYL STARLING, California Department of Public Health

*Orlando, New York, Chicago*
    TIA POWELL, Montefiore-Einstein Center for Bioethics

### Discussion with Attendees

## SESSION II: LOCAL AND STATE STANDARDS OF CARE PROTOCOLS

Session Objective: An interactive discussion with local, state, and regional officials about efforts to establish standards of care. Discuss implementation strategies and how these protocols were advanced to become operational entities in their respective communities. What are the current opportunities and barriers to facilitating improved implementation of protocols?

### Session Objectives and Background

*Irvine, Chicago*
    JOHN HICK, Hennepin County Medical Center, MN, *Session Chair*

*Orlando, New York*
    DAN HANFLING, Inova Health System, *Session Chair*

### Panel Discussion with State and Local Leaders

*Irvine*
    KAY FRUHWIRTH, Los Angeles County Emergency Medical Services
      Agency
    KRISTI KOENIG, University of California–Irvine
    PAUL PATRICK, State of Utah Department of Health
    SUSAN ALLAN, University of Washington School of Public Health
    CHRISTINE DENT, Saint Alphonsus Regional Medical Center, ID

*Orlando*
    JOHN ROBINSON, Baptist Memorial Hospital–North Mississippi
    ROY ALSON, North Carolina Office of Emergency Medical Services
    ROBERT HOOD, Florida Department of Health
    KENN BEEMAN, Mississippi State Department of Health

*New York*
    TIA POWELL, Montefiore-Einstein Center for Bioethics
    DONNA LEVIN, Massachusetts Department of Public Health
    LISA KAPLOWITZ, Alexandria Health Department, Virginia
    RICK HONG, Delaware Division of Public Health

*Chicago*
>JANET ARCHER, Indiana State Department of Health
>DAVID FLEMING, University of Missouri School of Medicine
>KERRY KERNEN, Summit County Health District, OH
>KEN BERKOWITZ, Veterans Health Administration National Center for Ethics in Health Care

## Response Panel

*Irvine*
>STEPHEN CANTRILL, Denver Health Medical Center
>JEFFREY DUCHIN, Public Health, Seattle and King County
>CHERYL STARLING, California Department of Public Health

*Orlando*
>STEPHEN CANTRILL, Denver Health Medical Center
>RADM ANN KNEBEL, Office of the Assistant Secretary for Preparedness and Response, U.S. Department of Health and Human Services
>JACK HERRMANN, National Association of County and City Health Officials

*New York*
>STEPHEN CANTRILL, Denver Health Medical Center
>CHERYL PETERSON, American Nurses Association

*Chicago*
>STEPHEN CANTRILL, Denver Health Medical Center
>CHERYL PETERSON, American Nurses Association
>TIA POWELL, Montefiore-Einstein Center for Bioethics

## Discussion with Attendees

- What resources, guidelines, and expertise have been used to establish standards of care protocols?
- What are the current opportunities and barriers to creating stronger partnerships and how can these issues be addressed?
- What strategies have been used to help integrate these protocols into practice?
- What are the current opportunities and barriers to facilitating improved implementation of protocols?

## SESSION III: PROVIDER COMMUNITIES

<u>Session Objective:</u> Discuss the roles and responsibilities of the key provider communities in the development and implementation of standards of care protocols. Identify and discuss solutions related to implementing protocols into practice.

### Session Objectives and Background

*Irvine, Orlando, New York, Chicago*
    STEPHEN CANTRILL, Denver Health Medical Center, *Session Chair*

### Panel Discussion with Stakeholder Leaders

*Irvine*
    SUE HOYT, St. Mary Medical Center, Long Beach, CA
    DEBRA WYNKOOP, Utah Hospitals and Health Systems Association
    ASHA DEVEREAUX, Sharp Coronado Hospital, CA
    KEVIN MCCULLEY, Association for Utah Community Health

*Orlando*
    J. PATRICK O'NEAL, Georgia Department of Human Resources
    KNOX ANDRESS, Louisiana Poison Center
    SHAWN ROGERS, Oklahoma State Department of Health
    LORI UPTON, Texas Children's Hospital
    MARY FALLAT, University of Louisville, KY

*New York*
    VALERIE SELLERS, New Jersey Hospital Association
    BRIAN CURRIE, Montefiore Medical Center
    CATHERINE RUHL, Association of Women's Health, Obstetric and
      Neonatal Nurses
    GEORGE FOLTIN, New York University School of Medicine/Bellevue
      Hospital

*Chicago*
    MICHAEL ROBBINS, Chicago Department of Public Health
    LESLEE STEIN-SPENCER, National Association of State EMS
      Officials

MARIANNE LORINI, Akron Regional Hospital Association
CONNIE J. BOATRIGHT, Managed Emergency Surge for Healthcare (MESH), IN

## Response Panel

*Irvine*

EDWARD GABRIEL, The Walt Disney Company
KATHRYN BRINSFIELD, Office of Health Affairs, Department of Homeland Security
MARGARET MCMAHON, Emergency Nurses Association

*Orlando*

EDWARD GABRIEL, The Walt Disney Company
KATHRYN BRINSFIELD, Office of Health Affairs, Department of Homeland Security
MARGARET MCMAHON, Emergency Nurses Association
CHERYL PETERSON, American Nurses Association

*New York*

JACK HERRMANN, National Association of County and City Health Officials
MARGARET MCMAHON, Emergency Nurses Association
CHERYL PETERSON, American Nurses Association

*Chicago*

JAMES J. JAMES, American Medical Association
MARGARET MCMAHON, Emergency Nurses Association
CHERYL PETERSON, American Nurses Association

## Discussion with Attendees

- What concerns do provider communities have in implementing policies into practice?
- How do protocols get implemented operationally?
  - Who is responsible for implementing plans during events?
  - What are the triggers?
- What action steps are required to improve involvement of the provider community in the development of standards of care protocols?

## SESSION IV: INTERSTATE AND NEIGHBORING COMMUNITY COOPERATION AND COORDINATION

Session Objective: Discuss what cooperation and coordination will be required between neighboring states and communities in preparation and when implementing standards of care protocols. Discuss the roles of specific stakeholders. Identify what resources will be required and how those may be shared. Explore the current opportunities and barriers to facilitating improved cooperation and coordination and how these may be overcome.

### Session Objectives and Background

*Irvine*
> CHERYL STARLING, California Department of Public Health, *Session Chair*

*Orlando*
> EDWARD GABRIEL, The Walt Disney Company, *Session Chair*

*New York*
> JACK HERRMANN, National Association of County and City Health Officials, *Session Chair*

*Chicago*
> SALLY PHILLIPS, Agency for Healthcare Research and Quality, *Session Chair*

### Panel Discussion with State and Local Leaders

*Irvine*
> NANCY AUER, Swedish Medical Center, WA
> MARK GOLDSTEIN, Memorial Health System, CO
> JEFFREY RUBIN, California Emergency Medical Services Authority

*Orlando*
> TERRY SCHENK, Florida Department of Health
> ROBERT BALL, South Carolina Department of Health and Environmental Control
> RAYMOND PEPE, Uniform Law Commission

*New York*
STEVEN GRAVELY, Troutman Sanders LLP
JAMES HODGE, Johns Hopkins University
FLOYD RUSSELL, West Virginia University
JAMES GEILING, White River Junction Veterans Administration
    Medical Center

*Chicago*
TIM WIEDRICH, North Dakota Department of Health
WILLIAM FALES, Michigan State University–Kalamazoo Center for
    Medical Studies
PAULA NICKELSON, Department of Health and Senior Services, MO
TIMOTHY CONLEY, Western Springs Fire Department and
    Emergency Medical Services, IL

## Response Panel

*Irvine*
DAN HANFLING, Inova Health System
SHAWN FULTZ, Department of Veterans Affairs
LTC(P) WAYNE HACHEY, Department of Defense
CAPT DEBORAH LEVY, Centers for Disease Control and Prevention

*Orlando*
DAN HANFLING, Inova Health System
SHAWN FULTZ, Department of Veterans Affairs
LTC(P) WAYNE HACHEY, Department of Defense
CAPT DEBORAH LEVY, Centers for Disease Control and Prevention
JAMES BLUMENSTOCK, Association of State and Territorial Health
    Officials

*New York*
DAN HANFLING, Inova Health System
RICHARD CALLIS, Department of Veterans Affairs

*Chicago*
DAN HANFLING, Inova Health System
DARLENE WEISMAN, Department of Veterans Affairs

## Discussion with Attendees

- What cooperation will be needed between states and neighboring communities?
- What are the roles of providers and other stakeholders in ensuring cooperation and coordination?
- How can resources best be shared during an event and what plans and agreements need to be in place?
- What strategies can be used to improve coordination and cooperation among neighboring jurisdictions?

## SESSION V: GENERAL DISCUSSION WITH WORKSHOP PARTICIPANTS AND ATTENDEES

Session Objective: Discuss what opportunities and constraints exist to implementing standards of care at local, state, and regional jurisdictions. Review opportunities and challenges identified during the workshop. Identify and discuss the most promising near-term opportunities for improving standards of care protocols at local, state, and regional jurisdictions. Discuss common threads that emerged among each of the regional workshops.

### Synopsis of Today's Discussions: Common Threads

SALLY PHILLIPS, Agency for Healthcare Research and Quality, *Workshop Chair*

### Discussion with Attendees

- What new ideas have surfaced in this meeting today that should be explored further?
- What specific challenges arise in the development of standards of care protocols?
- What action steps are required to integrate these strategies into the current public health system?
- What resources and further infrastructure investments will be necessary in the short- and long-term?

# D

# Participant Feedback Survey Responses

Feedback surveys were sent to all registered attendees at the workshops. The questions and responses are shown below. The total number of responses for each question was 53, unless otherwise indicated.

## 1. Which workshop did you attend?

|                        | Count | Percentage |
|------------------------|-------|------------|
| Irvine, CA–March 12    | 8     | 15%        |
| Orlando, FL–April 14   | 20    | 38%        |
| New York, NY–April 27  | 10    | 19%        |
| Chicago, IL–May 8      | 15    | 28%        |

## 2. Which stakeholder group(s) do you represent? (Please choose all that apply)

|                             | Count | Percentage |
|-----------------------------|-------|------------|
| Healthcare provider         | 24    | 45%        |
| Emergency medical services  | 10    | 19%        |
| Emergency management        | 9     | 17%        |
| Hospital administration     | 9     | 17%        |
| First responder             | 6     | 11%        |
| Local health official       | 5     | 9%         |
| State health official       | 5     | 9%         |
| Professional association    | 4     | 8%         |
| Private sector              | 3     | 6%         |

|                                                              | Count | Percentage |
|--------------------------------------------------------------|-------|------------|
| Emergency communications dispatch services                   | 2     | 4%         |
| Academic                                                     | 1     | 2%         |
| Academic medicine; project for NYC Department of Health and Mental Hygiene | 1 | 2% |
| Community health center                                      | 1     | 2%         |
| Community health nurse                                       | 1     | 2%         |
| Federal agency representative                                | 1     | 2%         |
| Illinois Department of Public Health Emergency Response Coordinator | 1 | 2% |
| Local municipality                                           | 1     | 2%         |
| Metropolitan Medical Response System                         | 1     | 2%         |
| M.P.A. student                                               | 1     | 2%         |
| Medical Reserve Corps (MRC)                                  | 1     | 2%         |
| National Library of Medicine project; hospital medical library | 1   | 2%         |
| University professor                                         | 1     | 2%         |
| World network private sector/first responder                | 1     | 2%         |

NOTE: Percentages add to greater than 100 because some participants checked multiple groups.

## 3. Does the organization you represent have policies in place for "standards of care during a mass casualty event"?

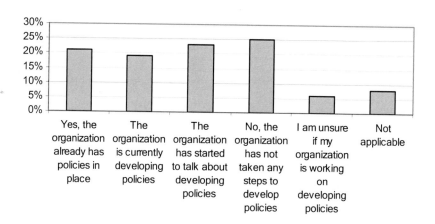

**4. Prior to the workshop, how familiar were you with the issues related to "standards of care during a mass casualty event" and with the work that has been done on this topic?**

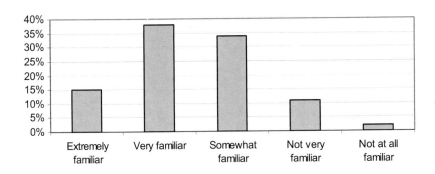

**5. How much work have you done developing or implementing policies related to the topic of "standards of care during a mass casualty event"?**

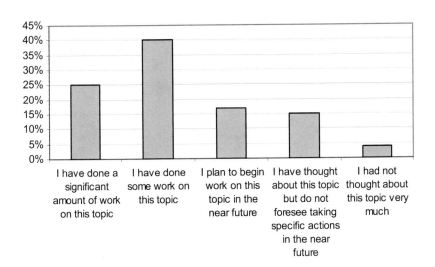

**6. Overall, how useful did you find the workshop in raising awareness of issues related to the topic of "standards of care during a mass casualty event"?**

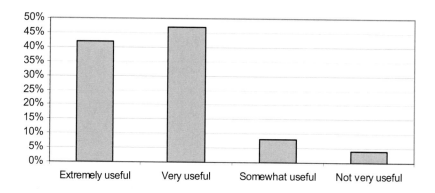

## (Optional) Comments

- A lot of useful information was brought up at the workshop, but it seemed as though attendance beyond people who sat on panels was quite limited. It would be useful to encourage attendance by stakeholders who are not a part of the formal presentations.

- We're preaching to the choir. We need to be explaining these issues to the general public.

- I found the most valuable portion of the workshop, for me, to be the beginning, when the focus was still on altered standards of care. When that focus was later lost, the workshop became less valuable for me.

- It was great at raising awareness, but not at answering the problems.

- Good questions posed by audience participants.

- I think the answer to this question is very dependent upon individual exposure.

- Lots of info, many propositions, even more questions left unanswered. Policies are new to all!

- All participants were well versed in the matter and provided outstanding insights to build upon.

- I was able to bring the technology issue into the debate, where it was not previously rated as important enough to be listed as a workgroup topic.
- It is important to hear other perspectives on the topic. Good to know others are struggling with similar issues.
- I think the topic of communication among agencies and communities would be a great topic for [a] workshop in the future.

**Total responses to this question: 11**


**7. What information presented or discussed during the workshop did you find most helpful?**

**[Sorted by response to Question 4: Prior knowledge]**

**Prior knowledge: Extremely or very familiar with issues**

- Overviews of various organizations and their interactions, especially the Florida planning.
- The idea of the continuum of standards to crisis care.
- "Rationing" and setting standards versus keeping one standard and identifying the shortcomings.
- "Lessons learned" discussions from panelists plus the Q and A.
- Policies and procedures developed by other states as noted in the resource files.
- "Disaster ethics"/bioethics discussion(s).
- That we are all struggling to apply ethical principles of fairness and justice within standards that we are developing across the United States.
- Medical ethics.
- The enlightenment of the subject being taboo at all levels.
- The importance of message during a mass casualty event, the importance of interjurisdictional license suspensions, and liability indemnification.
- So many it would be unfair to choose.
- Controversies surrounding rationing.
- Too many to identify them all. Developing the ethic platform for a state standard. Implementing altered standards of care through

emergency operations centers (EOCs) versus not (ND model).

- Views from all over the region.
- Surge capacity breakdown into three categories; rationing of scarce resources.
- Ethics issues.
- The need to educate the docs in the trenches.
- The discussions regarding the altered standards of care systems and to learn my local health department is not at the table. I understand the role the state health department plays; however, I feel that the LPHA has much more experience working with and within the local community than the state does.

**Total responses to this question: 18**

## Prior knowledge: Somewhat or not very familiar with issues

- The diversity of issues and approaches.
- Triage process.
- How expectations for care, along with the way we define good standards of care, must change in response to a mass casualty event.
- Discussion [of] the questions/issues that need to be addressed on the local level—and strategies for creating regional/national guidelines.
- Specifically what will be done, how, and by whom . . . protocol of hierarchy still needs more definition . . . and specific info as to resources and mass prophylaxis or actions.
- Ethics of group selection, the standards proposed by the VA.
- The concept of "rationing" equipment, care, and access.
- The information about getting state to state recognition as an EMT. The [H1N1] flu information was a touch-and-go subject that I thought I would love to get more information or education about.
- Interstate and neighboring community cooperation.
- Local and state standards.
- Discussions among presenters and attendees, and discussions with individuals during the break.

- Ethical principles and their application to mass casualty events. How individual facilities and regions are handling this issue.
- I was only able to attend the afternoon sessions . . . Session IV was outstanding . . . particularly Tim Conley, who related directly to municipality planning.
- That everyone is facing the same problem and that there is no "one" solution to the question. It will depend on local resources.
- The presentation on the need for coordination [among] various communities and sectors.
- SOFA + criteria for vents, who will be seen/admitted to the hospital during a pandemic. I was most impressed by the work of some of the state and regional groups.
- The overall discussion/definition of the topic was beneficial. The difficulties involved and general ideas of where the topic is headed were all helpful in determining how to help my organization respond.
- Discussion of surge capacity classification and Tia Powell's comments on the ethics of ventilator triage.

**Total responses to this question: 18**


**8. How will you use that information?**
**[Sorted by response to Question 4: Prior knowledge]**

**Prior knowledge: Extremely or very familiar with issues**

- Will use the notes from the workshop to start focus group discussions in many forums around the state to formulate the process for our state.
- Discuss with key hospital staff who will be involved with establishing altered standards of care and community emergency operations staff. Much of the info gathered from this conference will be included on hospital disaster preparedness webpage.
- Will adapt those to our Medical Reserve Corps component in Marion County, FL.
- Qualify current policy and procedures.
- Presentation to intradisaster response team to stimulate discussion on a topic that—perhaps—has been treated too incidentally.

- Serves as the foundation for further work at the local level.
- Will bring into our discussion locally.
- I will incorporate the information into telemedicine and apply it to the possible pandemic. The current reaction to the prepandemic is clearly a warning about preparedness for a pandemic event.
- Working with state agencies.
- Take topic to local and state committees dealing with pediatrics.
- I will report to the Oklahoma state committee on Altered Standards of Care much of what I absorbed.
- To take a second look at a couple of areas in our guidance. Appeals, triage officer.
- To begin discussion and development of policies to address these issues and to lobby the state Department of Public Health to do the same.
- Will activate in our Hospital Incident Command System (HICS) structure and proactively work with our ethics officer to help them prepare for disasters.
- Enhance our education program.
- If the goal is to be consistent, transparent, and fair, the local public health authority (LPHA) needs to be a part of the planning that is currently taking place if LPHAs are expected to assist in some sort of capacity.

**Total responses to this question: 16**

## Prior knowledge: Somewhat or not very familiar with issues

- Initiate further discussion in our region.
- Will educate providers on possible roles and decisions required during a disaster.
- I have raised the issue at our management discussions, and will continue to encourage that we do more practicing to prepare our response to a catastrophic event.
- My hospital needs to work on this—and we need to work on it as a region with other hospitals. Not sure that we will have much state input.
- I hope to use the information in a project on the legal aspects of

altered standards of care.

- To tell all my coworkers, friends, and family . . . send out an alert for the need to prepare for any catastrophic event.
- Discuss this with our county planning committee.
- Will use triage guidelines in our walk-in clinic/urgent care setting, and telephone triage guidelines for call-in questions.
- To continue my education and to assist others in other states in disasters as well as . . . our own state of New York.
- Bring ideas to my organization.
- Hope to follow up with individuals.
- Will work to develop policies with the American College of Surgeons and with our local community.
- It always reinvigorates me to attend anything on preparedness . . . I wish I would have been able to attend the morning sessions. I will take back to our regional group info. I received as well as shared it with our over 100 MRC members.
- To help initiate additional communication in the planning process for emergencies.
- I plan to start dialogue with our municipal fire department on issues heard at the workshop and attempt to [have a] dialogue with the supervisor and trustee of the township regarding the same.
- Keep my organization involved in the decision-making process with our regulating agencies.
- As a framework for further discussions.

**Total responses to this question: 17**

**9. Overall, how useful did you find the workshop in identifying practical solutions to some of the challenges you are facing in developing and implementing policies for "standards of care during a mass casualty event"?**

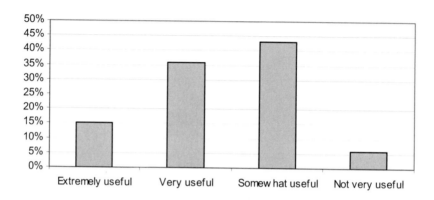

## (Optional) Comments

- Really are no "practical solutions" yet, really new untalked-about topic.
- Essentially, there are no answers anyone can give right now—but this brought to light all the important issues that need to be addressed.
- Format was excellent! Facilitated exchange of a large amount of information.
- [It did not provide many practical solutions . . .] but, it was excellent in raising the issues that need to be solved.
- We need to get more "in the weeds" and discuss things like disaster charting, contingency planning, etc.
- Policies in place are still in their draft stage; until a more permanent issuance occurs it is difficult to take action of any kind, meanwhile examples of other states' drafts help!
- I wish there was a protocol course that was mandatory for all EMTs and above to take for hands-on tactics or at least directed in the right direction for such. There should also be refresher courses for something such as disasters here and in other states.

- I think it's important to exchange ideas to formulate new or refine existing concepts.
- As expected at this type of event—more questions than answers!
- The Interstate Disaster Medical Cooperative (IDMC) group was one practical effort discussed that I think has the potential to impact every community.

**Total responses to this question: 10**

**10. If applicable, please describe any practical solutions the workshop helped you to identify, and briefly describe the next actions you will take.**

**[Sorted by response to Question 5: Prior work]**

**Prior work: Have done a significant amount or some work on this topic**

- Don't have to reinvent the wheel. Good contacts and references to learn from.
- This workshop has validated many of the concerns shared by licensed healthcare providers in our area (FL). However, the policy makers and regulators in our state have not provided a forum for discussion and input from those in the trenches; perhaps this is something we can work on.
- Use of quantifiable scoring systems to determine priorities in provision of vaccines and antivirals in a pandemic.
- Policies need to pay particular attention to inclusive language, [that is,] consider population dynamics and demographics.
- We need to have much more of a discussion with our communities. The public cannot have expectations of a usual standard of care in an extreme event that results in such an impact on capacity and capabilities to provide that care.
- I think the workshop is a bit too esoteric and the panel's thought process needs to be more focused on operationalizing the basic concepts.
- Would like to have seen the conference a little more policy specific related to hospitals and redelegating roles to unlicensed personnel, and more about how and what to do just-in-time training.

The conference was very broad and not user specific enough. . . .

- I will move forward on the expenditure of $3 billion in the buildout of WNIS infrastructure in NYS with anticipation of a useful outcome if the pandemic should evolve into a major mass casualty, which is unclear as yet. The area of concentration will be to extend primary care into the community and minimize the assemblage of people around one or more infectious carriers in what a local hospital calls an alternate care area; to me it is an inoculation center and should be avoided. I find it especially risky to draw in potential carriers into close contact with patients with other illnesses, which may be impairing their ability to evoke an effective immune response. The expenditure will, in the current financial condition, require the assistance of the Federal Reserve to facilitate the issuance of debt directly or thru a participating primary dealer of the Federal Reserve System. The provisioning of funds will allow the purchase of empty St. John's Hospital and Mary Immaculate Hospital in Queens, NYC, from bankruptcy court and the provisioning of those facilities for a possible increase in patient population.
- Meeting with stakeholders to develop consensus.
- Developing our philosophical statement, including the ethical platform. Ideas for implementing altered standards of care via governor's Executive Order at the time of crisis and implementing via the state EOC versus working through the state legislature to pass language.

**Total responses to this question: 10**

**Prior work: Had not done any work on this topic**

- Work with staff to create policies/procedures.
- Further workshop, stay informed and current. . . .
- I found there were people there that pointed me in the right direction on how to obtain a state-to-state registry, but what I can't understand is why does not every state acknowledge this (NREMS) and why is there yet ANOTHER charge for taking the test for the first time?
- Tools with their limitations for rationing scarce resources. Tools to begin the discussion with leadership.

- We need to really address standards of care. I will contact our local CCDPH rep. concerning this and request guidelines that I can share with neighboring communities, as well as my own.
- The effort [made by] the IDMC, spoken of by Tim Conley, is something I am going to look into to make sure my municipality is participating in.

**Total responses to this question: 6**

**11. Overall, how useful did you find the workshop in facilitating dialogue and relationships among stakeholders?**

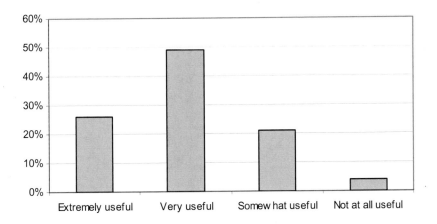

**(Optional) Comments**

- I imagine it was more useful for the other people there who are from the same area.

- I learned a great deal from the various experts. I was most disappointed that FL Board of Medicine and Nursing, Agency for Health Care Administration, and Emergency Management were not active participants. Lines of authority among these agencies once an emergency has been declared need to be established, especially among public and private healthcare providers who may have to resort to some form of altered standards of care. At present there is little interface.

- Networking opportunities were tremendous. Would have liked more time to speak with other participants.

- I greatly appreciated the significance of ongoing dialogues as noted above. However, my situation demands dialogues and communication within our institution, as well as without. I am concerned about these internal communications issues, as well.

- I have made some important contacts and hope others have gained some insight.

- I was sorry that more people were not able to attend due to H1N1 or other reasons.

- Networking is always most helpful.

- The dialogue that ensued was most interesting and informative, particularly hearing different viewpoints from different areas of expertise.

**Total responses to this question: 8**

**12. If applicable, please elaborate on how the workshop helped (or will help) you to develop relationships among stakeholders.**

- Good sound structure given for basic and advanced networking.

- Listening to the panel discussions helped to raise awareness of the many different types of scenarios.

- I was pleased to be able to meet others who are working in this area, and anticipate that now knowing them will be of great value to us in our anticipated project on legal issues involving altered standards of care.

- I made contact with some stakeholders, and hopefully plans for networking will materialize.

- It's always interesting to hear differing opinions. Requesting clarification on those "differing opinions" allows us to better understand and therefore work more synergistically with one another should the need arise.

- It was great to meet other "like minds" who are interested in this topic. I liked the way there was a panel of presenters on each topic.

- My actions are dictated by my position as an MRC member.

- It was very informative and will help to get the information that I have learned out to others, including other EMTs and higher that I work with.

- I will maintain ongoing communication during mass casualty events.

- Ability to know who individuals are, more than presentation content, which was quite rushed.

- I became aware of experts in this area and who needs to be included in efforts to develop guidelines.

- It always helps to put faces with names and begin to establish personal relationships with others concerned about the same issues.

- I collected business cards from those states that were developing similar frameworks to Oklahoma.

- Developed contacts in Illinois that will help with crossborder issues.

- Although I knew many of the attendees, it is always helpful to hear this discussion together. And it is helpful to give feedback to the presenters.

- I will need to meet with our local hospitals (one was represented at this workshop) and learn what their particular standards of care are in an emergency.

- It helped me to identify the areas where we need to work on building relationships. Two such are with residents and doctors.

- The workshop offered a forum with some "familiar local faces" that I now know are involved and can partner with as well as introducing new organizations/individuals that I can reach out to.

**Total responses to this question: 19**

**13. Is there anything else you would like to tell the workshop planning committee, for example:**

- **About issues that you did not feel were sufficiently addressed during the workshop?**
- **About next actions you intend to take on this topic?**
- **About the organization of the workshop?**

---

- Will use the available links and resources for additional help and info.

- Bring the Trial Lawyers of America on board.

- I would like to have the opportunity to work with some of those who presented in the workshop when we begin our project on legal issues related to altered standards of care. Thank you for putting on this workshop and for giving us the opportunity to be involved.

- (1) There needs to be transparency/accountability for federal funding; tracing the money has been impossible once it is released to the state (FL). Application/distribution/results of this funding are also a mystery. (2) Interface among county health departments, emergency management, and healthcare facilities and providers is weak. There is confusion about lead authority and roles/responsibilities. (3) Liability issues for healthcare providers/facilities have not been adequately addressed. (4) Suggestion for next workshop topic: View from the Trenches. It is my belief that there is not enough exchange of info between these levels and we could be missing some important issues/lessons. Next action: We will be meeting with hospital and community leaders to frame/discuss these issues and try to engage state officials. The panelists and experts were excellent sources of information, but as I stated on previous answers, the lack of participation by professional boards/regulators and public health preparedness from FL was quite troubling. Thank you for the opportunity to participate in the workshop and survey. Keep up the good work.

- Minimal attention was paid to the relatively large psychological footprint of a multicasualty disaster, especially to the value of group crisis intervention when staff [are] limited. Individual psychological first aid would be quite impractical in large-scale incidents.

- Great job presenting the issues and bringing the stakeholders together.

- I thought it was done overall very well.

- It was time well spent. A few folks seemed to use the time to "vent," which is fine—there is nothing wrong with expressing a real concern over an important issue or frustration; however, at times it seemed redundant. After the worries are expressed, we should concentrate on solutions.

- Need a clinical workshop directed at the operational side of provision of care during an extreme event. This workshop could provide guidelines for the evidence base to support contingency planning when resources are scarce.

- More workshops with the experts in the field are extremely satisfying.

- Future workshops should utilize speakers who are focused on the issues, not focused on their personal accomplishments or showing off their vocabulary.

- Have the next event posted on listservs for American College of Physicians, American College of Emergency Physicians, and other professions.

- I would like to see someone come out with a better way to bring all the states together so that certification would not be so difficult to get and not only in disasters. I feel that if we as emergency medical services give of ourselves in disasters/mass casualties and we are recognized then, we should be recognized nationally without having to take other exams. If we are capable at those times, is it not feasible that we are just as capable when there is not?

- I think a separate committee must be established to coordinate the development of e-tel nursing medicine as a viable intervention in mass casualty events. I will chair such a committee.

- I felt the presentations were hurried; I'm not sure what solutions exist to this problem other than follow-up information, notes, etc., that will be provided.

- No, it was well designed, attended, and implemented.

- Too much emphasis on bio events, which is understandable as the participants were mainly public health and government agency types who work in bio fields. But bio events are real outliers in the realm of disasters, being one of the least likely mass casualty scenarios and having a prolonged time course unlike virtually all other forms of disaster. [They] give time for surge to develop and to discuss altered standards that most disasters do not, as most disasters occur immediately with immediate overwhelming of resources with no warning—there is no progression from conventional to contingency to crisis over days to weeks in most disasters—it is conventional to crisis in 15 minutes. And therefore some of the issues and challenges, especially the time constraints and chaos. are quite different. An honest effort must be made in meetings such as these to broaden the perspective and understand that as important as bio events are to prepare for, their actual level of threat is quite low—look at history and read the newspapers to see what threats face us everyday. The feds and the AMA and CDC must get themselves out of this fixation on bio while ignoring the more likely scenarios. Ethical and moral and medical issues cut across all disasters and should not be just applied to influenza pandemics.

- Pediatrics always needs more emphasis, since 25 percent of the population in the United States is children; people are developing tools (Akron, OH, for example), but then "they are not applicable for children." It was helpful to hear the debate on whether scoring tools developed for adults can be transferred to children. The organization of the workshop was easy to follow and helpful to obtain a wide perspective. The audience participation was also useful. I only wish a number of my colleagues could have participated.

- I would have benefited from more discussion regarding the different states' strategies to actually implement their altered standards of care within the political climate of their state. For example, MO has made progress, but has a new governor. If the state is relying on a governor's Executive Order, what happens with a new governor? Are any states trying to pass language within the state legislature?

- We could have talked all day on this topic! Perhaps more time for just open discussion.

- Please find ways to engage the physician stakeholders.

- Thank you!

- I would have liked to hear how EMS Incident Command will interact.

- It was a very interesting workshop. I am not sure if I will use the info, but it was reassuring to know that we are on the right track in our planning.

- The organization was excellent!

- Thank you to the AMA for hosting the workshop and to the IOM for making it available to those of us in the community.

- Overall, I was very impressed with the workshop planning and facilitation. I would like to see continued follow-up information and contact (such as this survey) to maintain channels of communication. The workshops offered a method of outreach to regional, state, and local participants and I would encourage you to cultivate those contacts.

- It would have been helpful to better understand the IOM's eventual overall goals with defining standards of care in a mass casualty event. Will a guideline be published as a result of these workshops? The frustrating thing is that so many efforts are happening on many different levels, and I feel that there is much reinventing the wheel going on that might be unnecessary. I was hoping this workshop would help in outlining general accepted standards to be adopted and supported everywhere.

**Total responses to this question: 28**

# E

# Biographical Sketches of Workshop Planning Committee Members, Invited Speakers, and Panelists

## WORKSHOP PLANNING COMMITTEE

**Sally Phillips, Ph.D., R.N.** (*Chair*), currently serves as the director of the Agency for Healthcare Research and Quality (AHRQ) Public Health Emergency Preparedness Program. Dr. Phillips joined the staff of AHRQ's Center for Primary Care, Prevention, and Clinical Partnerships in 2001 as a senior nurse scholar. She managed a portfolio that ranged from her primary area of bioterrorism to multidisciplinary education for safety and related healthcare workforce initiatives. Prior to joining AHRQ, Dr. Phillips was a Robert Wood Johnson Health Policy Fellow and health policy analyst for Senator Tom Harkin for 2 years. She brought a wealth of expertise in the areas of multidisciplinary education, patient safety legislative initiatives, and curriculum with health professions education to her role at AHRQ. Dr. Phillips joined the AHRQ staff in 2002 as director of the Bioterrorism Preparedness Research Program, now the Public Health Emergency Preparedness Program. She is an accomplished author, consultant, and speaker on public health and medical preparedness and response research initiatives. Dr. Phillips holds a Ph.D. from Case Western Reserve University.

**James Blumenstock, M.A.,** holds the position of chief program officer for public health practice for the Association of State and Territorial Health Officials (ASTHO). His portfolio includes the state public health practice program areas of infectious and emerging diseases, immunization, environmental health, and public health preparedness and security, including pandemic influenza preparedness. Mr. Blumenstock also serves as a member of the ASTHO's Executive Management Team responsible for enterprise-wide strategic planning, administrative services, member support, and public health advocacy. Prior to his arrival at ASTHO in 2005, Mr. Blumenstock was the deputy commissioner of health for the New Jersey Department of Health and Senior Services, where he retired after nearly 32 years of career public health service. In this capacity, he had executive oversight responsibilities for a department branch of more than 650 staff and an operating budget of approximately $125 million. He oversaw the Division of Public Health and Environmental Laboratories; Division of Epidemiology, Occupational and Environmental Health; Division of Local Health Practice and Regional Systems Development; Division of Health Emergency Preparedness and Response; and the Office of Animal Welfare. During his tenure, Mr. Blumenstock also represented the department on a number of boards, councils, and commissions including the New Jersey Domestic Security Preparedness Task Force. Mr. Blumenstock is the proud recipient of the ASTHO 2004 Noble J. Swearingen Award for excellence in public health administration and the Dennis J. Sullivan Award, the highest honor bestowed by the New Jersey Public Health Association for dedicated and outstanding service and contribution to the cause of public health. He is also a Year 14 Scholar of the Public Health Leadership Institute and held an elected office serving his community for 12 years. He received his B.S. in Environmental Science from Rutgers University in 1973 and his M.A. in Health Sciences Administration from Jersey City State College in 1977.

**Katie Brewer, M.S.N., R.N.,** is a senior policy analyst with the American Nurses Association (ANA). Her areas of focus are public health infrastructure, including immunization, disaster preparedness and response, emerging disease, and public health workforce. Prior to joining ANA, Ms. Brewer practiced public health nursing with the Arlington County, VA, health department, serving as the county's immunization clinical services coordinator and playing key roles in public health communication efforts. She was involved in planning for and participating in public health emergency response exercises, as well as serving in incident command roles in actual emergencies. Ms. Brewer received her B.S.N. from Columbia University and her M.S.N. in Systems Management from the University of Virginia.

**Kathryn Brinsfield, M.D., M.P.H., FACEP,** is the associate chief medical officer for Component Services. She joined the U.S. Department of Homeland Security (DHS) Office of Health Affairs in 2008 to serve as operational and medical support medical director. Dr. Brinsfield left Boston as an associate professor of Boston University's Schools of Medicine and Public Health, with 13 years of experience as an attending physician at Boston City Hospital/Boston Medical Center. She graduated with honors from Brown University, received her M.D. from Tufts School of Medicine, and her M.P.H. from Boston University. She completed her residency in Emergency Medicine at Cook County Hospital in Chicago, and her emergency medical services (EMS) fellowship at Boston EMS. She has held medical director/associate medical director positions in various organizations, including Boston Emergency Services, Boston Homeland Security, and Boston Public Health Preparedness. She chaired the American College of Emergency Physicians' (ACEP's) Disaster Committee; cochaired the Massachusetts State Surge Committee; helped to create the Massachusetts Alternate Standards of Care Committee; and was commander of the Massachusetts-1 Disaster Medical Assistance Team and a supervisory medical officer for the International Medical and Surgical Response Team, which responded to the September 11, 2001, attacks.

**Stephen Cantrill, M.D., FACEP,** is an emergency physician from Denver who recently retired from serving as the associate director of emergency medicine at Denver Health Medical Center for 18 years. He was also director of the Colorado BNICE WMD Training Program at Denver Health for more than 5 years. Dr. Cantrill has lectured nationally and internationally on many topics, including weapons of mass destruction, disasters, and disaster management, and has been involved in disaster management education for more than two decades. He served as the regional medical coordinator for Denver's participation in Operation TOPOFF 2000. He has also been involved in weapons of mass destruction training for Colorado and has participated in the planning for multiple mass gathering events, including the Denver Papal visit and the Denver Summit of Eight world economic conference. He has testified at U.S. Senate Committee hearings on bioterrorism preparedness. He recently served as the principal investigator on an AHRQ regional surge capacity grant and the AHRQ National Hospital Available Beds for Emergencies and Disasters (HAvBED) project. He also served as principal investigator on the AHRQ disaster alternate care facility task order.

Dr. Cantrill has more than 90 publications and has been the recipient of multiple teaching and clinical excellence awards.

**CAPT D. W. Chen, M.D., M.P.H.,** is the director of Civil–Military Medicine in the Office of the Assistant Secretary of Defense for Health Affairs. Dr. Chen was the director of the Human Health Sciences Division, Office of Public Health and Science, Food Safety and Inspection Service. He previously served as director of the Division of Transplantation for the U.S. Department of Health and Human Services (HHS), which regulates the nation's organ and tissue transplant system. At HHS, he also worked in medical education and public health workforce development. Dr. Chen is an active duty commissioned officer with the U.S. Public Health Service. He is board certified in Preventive Medicine and a Fellow of the American College of Preventive Medicine. He completed his undergraduate studies at Harvard University, and earned his M.P.H. from the Harvard School of Public Health and his M.D. from Tufts University School of Medicine.

**Jeffrey Duchin, M.D.,** is chief of the Communicable Disease Control, Epidemiology & Immunization Section for Public Health, Seattle and King County, WA, and associate professor of medicine, Division of Infectious Diseases at the University of Washington. He holds appointments as adjunct associate professor in the schools of Public Health and Community Medicine and Health Services, and as faculty, Northwest Center for Public Health Practice. He is also the director of emergency response for the Northwest Regional Center of Excellence in Biodefense and Emerging Infectious Disease Research. Dr. Duchin trained in internal medicine at Thomas Jefferson University Hospital followed by a fellowship in general internal medicine and emergency medicine at the Hospital of the University of Pennsylvania. He did his infectious disease subspecialty training at the University of Washington. He is a graduate of the Centers for Disease Control and Prevention's (CDC's) Epidemic Intelligence Service, assigned to the National Center for Infectious Diseases, during which time he received the Outstanding Unit Citation for exemplary performance of duty, the Secretary's Recognition Award for exceptional performance in the investigation of unexplained deaths associated with an outbreak of acute illness of unknown etiology in the Four Corners area of the southwestern United States, and the Achievement Medal, HHS. Dr. Duchin subsequently worked for CDC as a medical epidemiologist in the Divisions of Tuberculosis Elimination and

HIV/AIDS Special Studies Branch before assuming his current position. He is a Fellow of the American College of Physicians and of the Infectious Disease Society of America (IDSA), where he chairs the IDSA's Bioemergencies Task Force and is a member of the Pandemic Influenza Task Force. He acts as liaison between the National Association of City and County Health Officials (NACCHO) and CDC's Advisory Committee on Immunization Practices. Dr. Duchin was a member of the HHS 2004 Tiger Team consulting with the government of Greece on health preparations for the 2004 Olympics in Athens. Since 1999, when the World Trade Organization Ministerial came to Seattle, he has been working to strengthen the ties among public health, clinicians, and the healthcare delivery system and to improve the response of the healthcare system and clinicians to public health emergencies, including biological terrorism and pandemic influenza. He is active in local, regional, and national preparedness planning activities for communicable disease emergencies, recently including pandemic influenza. Dr. Duchin's peer review publications and research interests focus on communicable diseases of public health significance, and he has authored text book chapters on the epidemiology of HIV/AIDS, bioterrorism, and outbreak investigations.

**Edward Gabriel, M.P.A., AEMT-P,** is director, Global Crisis Management, for The Walt Disney Company. He is responsible for the development and implementation of global policy, planning, training, and exercises to manage crisis for The Walt Disney Company. He is also responsible for East and West Coast Medical and Emergency Medical Operations and The Walt Disney Studio's Fire Department. He supports and collaborates with global business units in development and testing of resumption planning, and develops policies and strategies to manage crisis. Mr. Gabriel has been an Emergency Medical Technician (EMT) since 1973 and is a 27-year paramedic veteran of New York City Fire Department's EMS. He rose through the ranks from emergency medical technician (EMT) to paramedic through lieutenant, and retired at the level of assistant chief/division commander. As deputy commissioner for planning and preparedness at the New York City (NYC) Office of Emergency Management, he served as commissioner for all preparedness and planning-related projects and initiatives. During his role with New York City, he was a member of the Federal Bureau of Investigation/NYC Joint Terrorism Task Force, and still sits on the International Advisory Board of the *Journal of Emergency Care, Rescue and Transportation*. He has worked with The Joint Commission, sitting on the Emergency Preparedness Roundtable as well as the Community Linkages in Bioterrorism Preparedness Expert Panel. He served as a member of the HHS Federal Contingency Medical Facility Working Group and the AHRQ Expert Panel on Mass Casualty Medical Care. Most recently he has worked with the Expert Panel as principal author of the prehospital chapter of *Mass Medical Care with Scarce Resources: Community Planning Guide* and with the U.S. Department of Defense, General George C. Marshall School of International Studies Program on Terrorism and Security Studies, located in Garmisch-Partenkirchen, Germany, presenting on methodologies for planning and preparedness for international leaders. He is credentialed through the International Association of Emergency Managers as a Certified Emergency Manager (CEM) and the Disaster Recovery Institute International as a Certified Business Continuity Professional. Mr. Gabriel holds a B.A. from the College of New Rochelle and an M.P.A. from Rutgers University.

**LTC(P) Wayne Hachey, D.O., M.P.H.,** is the director of preventive medicine at the Office of the Deputy Assistant Secretary of Defense for Force Health Protection and Readiness, in the Office of the Assistant Secretary of Defense for Health Affairs. His background includes both nursing and medicine. He holds a B.S.N. and an M.S. in Pediatric Nursing. He earned his medical degree at Southeastern College of Osteopathic Medicine and an M.P.H. at the Uniformed Services University for Health Sciences (USUHS). He holds board certification in Pediatrics, Neonatal–Perinatal Medicine, and Preventive Medicine. He is responsible for developing preventive medicine and immunization policy affecting active-duty populations in the Department of Defense (DoD). He also serves as a subject-matter expert on pandemic/avian influenza. In the course of his duties, he has developed many of the DoD's medical policies and guidance regarding pandemic influenza, including the DoD's recent policy for prioritizing delivery of medical care during pandemics and other public health emergencies of national significance. He also serves as the DoD representative on a number of national pandemic and seasonal influenza planning committees. He represents the DoD in these subject areas in venues ranging from the White House to remote military clinics.

**Dan Hanfling, M.D.,** is special advisor to the Inova Health System in Falls Church, VA, on matters related to emergency preparedness and disaster response. He is a board-certified Emergency Physician practicing at Inova Fairfax Hospital, Northern Virginia's Level I trauma center. He serves as an operational medical director for PHI Air Medical Group–Virginia, the largest private rotor-wing air medevac service in Virginia. He has responsibilities as a medical team manager for Virginia Task Force One, an international urban search-and-rescue team sanctioned by the Federal Emergency Management Agency (FEMA) and the U.S. Agency for International Development (USAID). He has been involved in the response to international and domestic disaster events, including the response to the Izmit, Turkey, earthquake in 1999, the Pentagon in September 2001, the response to Hurricanes Rita and Katrina in 2005, and Gustav and Ike in 2008. Dr. Hanfling was intricately involved in the management of the response to the anthrax bioterror mailings in fall 2001, when two cases of inhalational anthrax were successfully diagnosed at Inova Fairfax Hospital. Dr. Hanfling received an A.B. in Political Science from Duke University and was awarded his M.D. from Brown University. He completed an internship in Internal Medicine at the Miriam Hospital in Providence, RI, and an Emergency Medicine Residency at George Washington/Georgetown University Hospitals. He is a clinical professor of emergency medicine at George Washington University and an invited member of the George Mason University School of Public Policy Advisory Board.

**Jack Herrmann, M.S.Ed., N.C.C., L.M.H.C.,** is the senior advisor for public health preparedness at NACCHO, an association that represents the approximately 3,000 local public health departments across the country. In this role, Mr. Herrmann oversees the organization's preparedness portfolio, which consists of five federally funded programs aimed at enhancing and strengthening the preparedness and response capacity of local health departments. He establishes the priorities for public health preparedness within the organization and also serves as the organization's liaison to local, state, and federal partner agencies. Prior to arriving to NACCHO, Mr. Herrmann was assistant professor of psychiatry and director of the Program in Disaster Mental Health at the University of Rochester Medical Center, Department of Psychiatry. Over his 17 years with the university, Mr. Herrmann brought a wealth of experience to the fields of disaster mental health, suicide prevention, and employee assistance program services. As the founder and former director of Strong EAP, Mr. Herrmann specialized in developing critical response teams for local police, fire, and healthcare organizations. He also developed a disaster mental health training curriculum, currently required training for behavioral health and spiritual care response teams throughout New York and Maine. Mr. Herrmann has also been a long-time volunteer with the American Red Cross. Since 1993, he has responded to numerous disasters, including the Northridge, CA, earthquake, the explosion of TWA Flight 800, and many hurricanes and floods. He was assigned as the mental health coordinator for the Family Assistance Center in NYC immediately following the September 11, 2001, attacks and also assisted the NYC Mayor's Office in coordinating the first and second year anniversaries of that event. In 2005 he was deployed as the client services administrator for the Hurricane Katrina relief operation (Louisiana), coordinating the health, mental health, and client casework services for the first 2 weeks following that storm. A month later he was deployed again to Louisiana in the same position following Hurricane Rita. In 2006, Mr. Herrmann responded to Lexington, KY, as the mental health manager following the crash of Comair Flight 5191. Mr. Herrmann earned a master's degree in Education from the University of Rochester, is certified by the National Board of Certified Counselors, and is a licensed mental health counselor in the state of New York.

**John L. Hick, M.D.,** is a faculty emergency physician at Hennepin County Medical Center (HCMC) and an associate professor of emergency medicine at the University of Minnesota. He serves as the associate medical director for Hennepin County Emergency Medical Services and medical director for emergency preparedness at HCMC. He is also medical advisor to the Minneapolis/St. Paul Metropolitan Medical Response System. He also serves the Minnesota Department of Health as medical director for the Office of Emergency Preparedness and as medical director for Hospital Bioterrorism Preparedness. He is the founder and past chair of the Minneapolis/St. Paul Metropolitan Hospital Compact, a 29-hospital mutual aid and planning group active since 2002. He is involved at many levels of planning for surge capacity and adjusted standards of care and traveled to Greece to assist its healthcare system preparations for the 2004 Summer Olympics as part of a 15-member CDC/HHS team. He is a national speaker on hospital preparedness issues and has published numerous papers dealing with hospital preparedness for contaminated casualties, personal protective equipment, and surge capacity.

**RADM Ann R. Knebel, R.N., D.N.Sc., FAAN,** is a registered nurse with a Doctorate of Nursing Science in Pulmonary Critical Care. For the past 16 years, she has served as an officer in the Public Health Service Commissioned Corps. Currently, she is deputy director for preparedness planning in the HHS Office of the Assistant Secretary for Preparedness and Response (ASPR). In this capacity she is responsible for the development of programs to enhance preparedness integration across the local/state/regional and federal tiers of response. In the 5 years Dr. Knebel has worked for ASPR (formerly the Office of Public Health Emergency Preparedness), she has been instrumental in advancing various preparedness planning and surge capacity initiatives. Currently she is leading a working group in coordination with FEMA to identify resource types for public health and medical teams to support state-to-state mutual aid. She was the HHS lead in assisting the Greek Ministry of Health to prepare for the 2004 Summer Olympics and completed a 9-month detail with the NYC Office of Emergency Management, developing bioterrorism plans. During the response to the 2005 hurricane season, Dr. Knebel worked as a chief planner on the HHS Emergency Management Team, helping to plan the federal public health and medical response and recovery. Prior to joining the ASPR, Dr. Knebel served in both the intramural and extramural programs at the National Institutes of Health (NIH). Activities included supporting clinical trials of the National Heart, Lung, and Blood Institute; conducting a research program on quality of life and symptom management in persons with genetic lung diseases; mentoring staff nurses in supporting biomedical research; and serving as a program director to build a portfolio in end-of-life research for the National Institute of Nursing Research. RADM Knebel responded to the first aid stations at the World Trade Center in response to the September 11, 2001, attacks and to the newly formed HHS Command Center during the anthrax attacks of 2001. She is a Fellow of the American Academy of Nursing.

**CAPT Deborah Levy, Ph.D., M.P.H.,** is a Captain with the U.S. Public Health Service and chief of the Healthcare Preparedness Activity in the Division of Healthcare Quality Promotion (DHQP) at the CDC. Captain Levy's primary focus is all-hazards healthcare preparedness and emergency response (including pandemic influenza, bioterrorism agents, and natural disasters such as hurricanes). She is currently focused on conducting cross-sector workshops on models of delivery of care at the community level, conducting healthcare stakeholder meetings to develop implementation tools, and working with medical societies to develop triage and clinical algorithms to deal with a surge in patients under conditions of scarce resources. She is overseeing cooperative agreements with nine states to determine essential healthcare services during an influenza pandemic. Captain Levy joined the CDC in 1996 as an epidemic intelligence service officer in the Division of Parasitic Diseases, where she focused on waterborne and foodborne diseases as well as water security issues before moving to CDC's DHQP in 2003. She earned a B.A. in Psychology and an M.P.H. in Epidemiology from the University of California–Los Angeles, and a Ph.D. in Epidemiology from Johns Hopkins University's Bloomberg School of Hygiene and Public Health.

**Anthony Macintyre, M.D.,** is a board-certified Emergency Physician and associate professor with the Department of Emergency Medicine at The George Washington University. His academic career has focused on medical emergency planning and response at various levels. Dr. Macintyre has served as the medical director for Fairfax County, VA's Urban Search and Rescue team since 1995. His work with the team has involved deployments to the bombing of the Murrah building in Oklahoma City (1995), the bombing of the U.S. Embassy in Nairobi (1998), the Pentagon terrorist attack (2001), and to several international earthquakes. His most recent deployment involved response to the devastating earthquake in Bam, Iran (2004), as part of the USAID team. Dr. Macintyre has assisted the FEMA (now part of the DHS) in the restructuring of the medical components of the Urban Search and Rescue System. Dr. Macintyre's work has also included assisting other U.S. federal agencies with medical emergency planning and response. He served as a medical advisor and a controller for the bioterrorism component of the federally sponsored exercise, TOPOFF 2000, held in Denver, CO. More recently, he served as an official observer of the Chicago component of TOPOFF 2003. In 2002, Dr. Macintyre served as an assistant investigator in the Sloan Foundation-funded project to develop the Medical and Health Incident Management system. This project provides a comprehensive, functionally based model for the response to and management of complex, large-scale medical emergencies. Dr. Macintyre was also the codeveloper of a mass decontamination capability for the old George Washington University Hospital (key concepts published in *JAMA*). In his capacity as an emergency physician, he was instrumental in structuring the hospital response to the 2001 anthrax dissemination event. Dr. Macintyre has served for 6 years on the District of Columbia Hospital Association Emergency Preparedness Committee, assisting with the development of a hospital community response for Washington, DC.

**Margaret (Peggy) M. McMahon, R.N., M.N., CEN,** is the editor of *Disaster Management & Response*, a journal of the Emergency Nurses Association (ENA), and is the emergency clinical nurse specialist at AtlantiCare Regional Medical Center–Mainland Campus in Pomona, NJ. She has more than 40 years of professional nursing experience in clinical, administrative, and educational settings, including active and reserve duty in the U.S. Army Nurse Corps, where she served as a nuclear, biological, and radiological defense officer. Ms. McMahon is a past president of the national ENA, and has lectured and published extensively on disaster and emergency care.

**Cheryl A. Peterson, M.S.N., R.N.,** is the director of nursing practice and policy at the American Nurses Association. Prior to that, she was a senior policy Fellow for the ANA, responsible for researching and developing association policy related to preparing for and responding to a disaster, whether man-made or natural. Since 1998, Ms. Peterson has been actively involved in disaster planning at the federal level. In addition, she coordinated the ANA's response to the tsunami disaster in Asia and to hurricanes during 2005. Ms. Peterson spent 13 years in the Reserve Army Nurse Corps, and in 1990 was deployed during Desert Storm. She also spent 7 years as an active volunteer in the Kensington (MD) Volunteer Fire Department. Ms. Peterson received her B.S.N. from the University of Cincinnati and her M.S.N. from Georgetown University.

**Tia Powell, M.D.,** is director of the Montefiore-Einstein Center for Bioethics and a faculty member at Albert Einstein College of Medicine and the Montefiore Medical Center in New York. She served from 2004 to 2008 as executive director of the New York State Task Force on Life and the Law and from 1992 to 1998 as director of clinical ethics at Columbia-Presbyterian Hospital in NYC. She is a graduate of Harvard-Radcliffe College and Yale Medical School. She did her psychiatric internship, residency, and a fellowship in Consultation-Liaison Psychiatry, all at Columbia University, College of Physicians and Surgeons, and the New York State Psychiatric Institute. She is a Fellow of the American Psychiatric Association and of the New York Academy of

Medicine and a member of the American Society of Bioethics and Humanities. In 2007, she cochaired the New York State Department of Health workgroup to develop guidelines for allocating ventilators during a flu pandemic.

**Cheryl Starling, R.N., M.S.,** is the pandemic influenza project director at the California Department of Public Health. She has more than 20 years of leadership experience in health care and emergency management preparedness, planning, and response. As a registered nurse and director of emergency departments and trauma centers across California for many years, Ms. Starling has broad experience in healthcare delivery, financing and budget, emergency medical services, ambulatory care services, quality management, and disaster preparedness. She recently served as threat assessment consultant for Kaiser Permanente, where she developed nationally recognized emergency management programs, and served as coexecutive director for the Center for the Hospital Incident Command System (HICS) Education and Training. Previously she led the statewide terrorism exercise for the California Homeland Security Training and Exercise Program.

**Eric Toner, M.D.,** is a senior associate with the Center for Biosecurity of the University of Pittsburgh Medical Center (UPMC). Dr. Toner is a widely cited author on a range of biosecurity issues, including hospital preparedness, pandemic influenza response, and clinical issues related to bioterrorism response. Dr. Toner has been involved in hospital disaster planning since the mid-1980s. Prior to joining UPMC, Dr. Toner was medical director of disaster preparedness at St. Joseph Medical Center in Towson, MD, and practiced emergency medicine for 23 years. During this time he also served as chief executive officer (CEO) and chief financial officer of a large group practice and as associate head of the Department of Emergency Medicine. He founded and directed one of the first Chest Pain Centers in Maryland. Dr. Toner also cofounded and managed a large primary care group practice and an independent urgent care center. After September 2001, he was appointed to the newly created position of medical director of disaster preparedness. He developed policies and procedures for decontamination, defense against respiratory pathogens, and surge capacity, and he had responsibility for biological, chemical, radiological, and nuclear preparedness issues, including preparedness and response for smallpox, severe acute respiratory system (SARS), and pandemic flu. He helped create a coalition of disaster preparedness personnel from the five Baltimore County hospitals, Health Department, and Office of Emergency Management. Dr. Toner received his B.A. and M.D. from the University of Virginia. He trained in Internal Medicine at the Medical College of Virginia. He is board certified in Internal Medicine and Emergency Medicine.

## INVITED SPEAKERS AND PANELISTS

**Susan Allan, M.D., J.D., M.P.H.,** has been the director of the Northwest Center for Public Health Practice since 2008. Prior to joining the University of Washington, she worked in state and local public health for more than 23 years, including 3 years as public health director and state health officer for Oregon, and 18 years as health director for Arlington County, VA. In those positions, she had gained experience with emergency preparedness, including responding to a wide range of actual emergencies and serving on many state and national emergency preparedness committees and workgroups. She is a member of the ASTHO Preparedness Policy Committee, and a Fellow of the American College of Preventive Medicine. She is also a member of the Board on Population Health and Public Health Practice of the Institute of Medicine, and is vice president of the Council on Education for Public Health.

**Roy L. Alson, Ph.D., M.D., FACEP,** began his EMT career in the 1970s as a responder. As a medical director in North Carolina EMS, he manages 800 firefighters, EMTs, and rescue personnel and over 20 agencies. He is an associate professor of emergency medicine at the Wake Forest University Baptist Medical Center, a Regional Level I Trauma Center and Burn Center. He received a bachelor's degree from the University of Virginia, and a Ph.D. and an M.D. from Bowman Gray School of Medicine of Wake Forest University. He completed a residency in Emergency Medicine at Allegheny General Hospital in Pittsburgh. He is certified by the American Board of Emergency Medicine, and is a Fellow of ACEP and American Academy of Emergency Medicine. He currently serves as medical director for Forsyth County EMS in North Carolina. He is the former commander and deputy commander of Disaster Medical Assistance Team (DMAT) NC-1 and has led the team's response to numerous disasters at the state and national levels, including Hurricanes Andrew and Katrina. He currently serves as the medical director for the

NC Office of EMS State Medical Response system. He serves on numerous committees and councils in various leadership roles, is active in nonprofit organizations, and is a contributing author to many texts.

**Knox Andress, R.N., FAEN,** is the director of emergency preparedness and education for the Louisiana Poison Center, within the Department of Emergency Medicine, Louisiana State University Health Sciences Center, Shreveport, LA. Mr. Andress previously was an emergency department (ED) and intensive care unit (ICU) nurse with the CHRISTUS Schumpert Health System in Shreveport for 14 years. During the past 3 years, he served as the hospital system's emergency preparedness coordinator, responsible for hospital disaster planning and education. He continues to serve on the CHRISTUS Health System's Emergency Management Council. Mr. Andress is the designated regional coordinator for Louisiana's 28 Region 7 hospitals coordinating bioterrorism and pandemic education, preparedness, and planning related to the Hospital Preparedness Program. During Hurricanes Katrina, Rita, Gustav, and Ike, Mr. Andress served as an incident commander in Louisiana's Region 7, Regional Hospital Coordinating Center, supporting hospital evacuations and patient movements into other hospitals and assisting with medical support for general and special needs shelters. He instructs and advises on a number of emergency department and hospital-related disaster management courses, including Hospital Incident Command System (HICS), multiple National Incident Management System (NIMS) courses, and Advanced HAZMAT Life Support. He serves as the "Hospital" subcommittee chair on the Altered Standards of Care committee of Louisiana's Clinical Pandemic Flu Forum. Mr. Andress has been a primary investigator benchmarking the evacuations of seven hospitals secondary to Hurricane Rita, studying the hurricane planning, impacts, and decision processes to evacuate. He is the ENA's Emergency Management and Preparedness Committee chair.

**Janet Archer, R.N., M.S.N.,** is the chief nurse consultant in the Public Health Preparedness and Emergency Response Division of the Indiana State Department of Health. She received her bachelor's degree in Nursing from Ball State University and her master's degree in Nursing at Indiana University in Indianapolis. She worked for 12 years in the Emergency Department of Community Hospital East in Indianapolis and was active with hospital emergency preparedness activities and educational programs for EMTs and paramedics. When DMATs were developed by the National Disaster Medical System (NDMS), Ms. Archer implemented the first team in Indiana—DMATIN1. She also brought crisis mental health counseling to Indiana with the first Critical Incident Stress Management Team in the state. Ms. Archer served for 10 years as the director of emergency medical services at the Indiana Convention Center and RCA Dome. She was appointed to the Marion County Local Emergency Planning Committee (LEPC) and served on that committee for 15 years. As a member of the LEPC, she cofounded the Marion County Hospital Hazardous Materials Committee to ensure that hospitals would be included in disaster planning. Ms. Archer has been with the Indiana State Department of Health since 2005, and has been chair of the Pandemic Influenza Education Committee since that time. She has made more than 150 pandemic influenza educational presentations to audiences throughout the state. She initiated the development of a pandemic influenza education toolkit for local health departments and hospitals to use as they educate their communities about pandemic influenza. That toolkit was selected for presentation at the national Public Health Preparedness Summit in 2008. Ms. Archer is currently cochair of the Altered Standards of Care Community Advisory Group. Over the past 2 years, this committee has drafted a guidance document for medical facilities to use during a pandemic to decide who gets care when resources are scarce.

**Nancy Auer, M.D.,** is an emergency medical physician who serves as special medical advisor to the CEO at Swedish Medical Center. She oversees the management of clinical research, international patient and physician services, and Swedish's Institutional Review Board. Dr. Auer has been at Swedish for more than 28 years, serving in various key positions, including chief medical officer, chief of staff, medical director of emergency services, and vice president of medical affairs. Recognized as one of the top emergency medicine physicians in the country, Dr. Auer was the first woman president of the ACEP. In 2001, she received ACEP's annual John G. Wiegenstein Leadership Award for being an inspirational, innovative leader with excellent management and decision-making skills. She was also elected an honorary member of ACEP for her outstanding service to the medical profession and to the college. She has served as president of the International Federation of Emergency Medicine and is past chair of the Emergency Medicine Foundation. She has also served as the medical director of the Seattle/King County Disaster Team since 1990 and is a past president of the Washington State

Medical Association (WSMA) and chair of WSMA's Executive Committee. Currently, she serves as chair of the board for the Washington Health Foundation. Dr. Auer also serves as volunteer medical director of bioterrorism planning for the state. Board certified in Emergency Medicine, Dr. Auer lectures often and has been published numerous times. Examples include her testimony before the U.S. Senate Judiciary Committee on the growing crisis of drug abuse among children, her chapter on emergency treatment of head injuries in the *National Medical Students Handbook of Emergency Medicine*, and her speech on "Women in Organized Medicine" to the Congress of Neurosurgery. In 2008, ACEP honored Dr. Auer with its Hero of Emergency Medicine award, which recognizes physicians who have made significant contributions to emergency medicine, their communities, and their patients. Dr. Auer is a graduate of the University of Chattanooga, where she was also a Teaching Fellow in the department of biology. She earned her M.D. from the University of Tennessee Medical School and completed her surgery internship in City of Memphis Hospitals. Her residency was done at the University of Tennessee Medical School. She received her leadership/management training at the Battelle Institute in Seattle.

**Robert T. Ball, Jr., M.D., M.P.H.,** is an infectious disease epidemiologist with the South Carolina Department of Health and Environmental Control, where he focuses on planning for pandemic influenza. Before joining the department, Dr. Ball practiced medicine for many years and diagnosed South Carolina's first AIDS case in 1982. Dr. Ball was involved in establishing the state's reporting system for HIV/AIDS and in guiding the state's initial response to the disease. In 1990 he led a team of health professionals and community advocates that designed a statewide plan to attack the AIDS epidemic. Dr. Ball earned his M.D. from Medical University of South Carolina and his M.P.H. from the University of South Carolina School of Public Health.

**S. Kenn Beeman, M.D., FACS,** is a senior physician assigned to the Office of Emergency Planning and Response within the Mississippi State Department of Health (MSDH). As a relative newcomer to the agency, his professional interest and preoccupation have revolved principally around pandemic influenza; to a lesser but still important extent, he has been intrigued with the impact of biomedical ethics on public health practice and planning, and engaged specifically with complementary strategies by which surge demand for acute care can be met with "adequate/sufficient" surge capacity in the midst of disasters. The latter involvement has manifested itself by nascent work with the development of a pediatric disaster network for Alabama and Mississippi, healthcare provider volunteerism, and the relatively new MSDH-based medical assistance teams. While his temperament frequently betrays the nature and identity of his former professional post, his rich and robust 13-year career in clinical cardiothoracic surgery at the North Mississippi Medical Center in Tupelo, MS, hardly represents the customary, well-traveled pathway to public health and population "medicine." A native Mississippian, he proudly lays claim to Ole Miss as his undergraduate alma mater. Upon receipt of his M.D. from the Vanderbilt University School of Medicine, he remained in Nashville for a split internship in Medicine and Pediatrics, before embarking on an academic residency in General Surgery under the auspices of the same institutions. His training culminated with a Fellowship in Cardiovascular and Thoracic Surgery at the Indiana University Hospitals in Indianapolis. He is a Fellow in the American College of Surgeons; volunteers with the local Good Samaritan Free Clinic in Tupelo; and participates in "organized medicine" matters in Mississippi. As a "summer-only" student in the "quantitative methods" concentration, Dr. Beeman is a candidate for the M.P.H. from the Harvard School of Public Health.

**Kenneth A. Berkowitz, M.D., FCCP,** is chief of ethics consultation at the VHA National Center for Ethics in Health Care. He also performs direct patient care and ethics-related activities at the NY Campus of the VA New York Harbor Health Care System and the New York University (NYU) School of Medicine. He is an internist specializing in pulmonary and critical care medicine, and he has additional clinical expertise in home care and end-of-life care. His career interest in medical ethics has focused on ethical health care practices, clinical and organizational ethics consultation, and ethics education. Dr. Berkowitz received his undergraduate degree in Biology from Brown University and his M.D. from Mount Sinai School of Medicine. He completed clinical training in Internal, Pulmonary, and Critical Care Medicine at the New York VA Medical Center and the NYU Medical Center. After his fellowship training, he joined the staff of the New York VA Medical Center and the faculty of the NYU School of Medicine, where he is now an associate professor of medicine. In 1996, he completed a Certificate Program in Bioethics and the Medical Humanities, sponsored jointly by the Columbia College of

Physicians and Surgeons and the Montefiore School of Medicine. He is now a visiting faculty member of the Certificate Program.

**James Blumenstock, M.A.,** *see Workshop Planning Committee biosketch.*

**Connie J. Boatright, M.S.N., R.N., COL, USAR (Ret.),** has served in emergency management in healthcare roles for more than 30 years. Since retiring as deputy director/acting director of the VA National Emergency Management Strategic Healthcare Group, Ms. Boatright has served as a subject matter expert (SME)/advisor to healthcare systems, hospitals, Community Health Centers (CHCs), and other entities. Recent assignments include SME consultant for the Managed Emergency Surge for Healthcare Coalition, a federal grant-supported program at the Department of Emergency Medicine, Indiana University School of Medicine, Indianapolis. She advises CHCs and Primary Care Associations, in areas such as Indiana and Washington, DC, and continues to serve on national emergency management task forces and committees, such as The George Washington University/VA Work Group on Emergency Management Programs and Credentialing. She also serves as faculty at the DHS's Noble Training Facility, Center for Domestic Preparedness, Anniston, AL. A recently retired U.S. Army Reserve Colonel, Ms. Boatright has published widely and presents frequently on emergency management in public health and healthcare systems. She is an advanced practice nurse and graduate of several military schools. Her background includes deployment to or in support of many presidentially declared disasters and events and service on national and international policy forums. In Ms. Boatright's honor, the VA has instituted the annual Connie J. Boatright Emergency Management Service Award, which recognizes an employee (from VA's nationwide system) who best exemplifies emergency management service excellence.

**Kathryn Brinsfield, M.D., M.P.H., FACEP,** *see Workshop Planning Committee biosketch.*

**Richard Callis, M.S.,** is deputy chief consultant for planning and operations with the Emergency Management Strategic Health Care Group at the VA. Previously, Mr. Callis was deputy superintendent of the Emergency Management Institute at FEMA. Prior to that, he served as the Integrated Emergency Management Section chief, stationed at the

Conference and Training Center, Mount Weather, VA. Mr. Callis has also served as the team leader for the Integrated Emergency Management Team and has managed the Professional Development Series of courses. Prior to joining federal service, he managed a state training program for 12 years and served as an instructor for a business management program for a private college. Mr. Callis has a B.S. in Business Administration and an M.S. in Education.

**Stephen Cantrill, M.D., FACEP,** *see Workshop Planning Committee biosketch.*

**Timothy Conley, EMT-P,** is the Director of Preparedness and Planning for the Village of Western Springs Department of Fire/EMS Services and Emergency Management. Mr. Conley's current duties also include H1N1 planning for the Village of Western Springs and Illinois Fire Service MABAS Division 10 (18 fire departments). He is also serving as a Planning Section Chief for the Missouri State Disaster Medical Team. Other relevent experience includes serving as the Team Commander and Management Support Team coordinator of the Illinois Medical Emergency Response Team, and as member of the Illinois Terrorism Task Force Bioterrorism and Pandemic flu committees.

**Brian P. Currie, M.D., M.P.H.,** is vice president/medical director for research at Montefiore Medical Center and assistant dean for clinical research at the Albert Einstein College of Medicine (AECOM). He is a graduate of the Albert Einstein College of Medicine and completed residency training in Internal Medicine at Bellevue Hospital/NYU and an Infectious Diseases Fellowship at AECOM/Montefiore Medical Center. Dr. Currie also received an M.P.H. in Epidemiology from the Columbia University School of Public Health. He has been on the faculty of the Albert Einstein College of Medicine for more than 15 years and has a joint appointment as professor of medicine and of epidemiology and population health. His academic interests include the application of molecular epidemiological methods to investigations of infectious diseases. In addition to his administrative responsibilities, Dr. Currie continues to practice and teach in the Division of Infectious Diseases at Montefiore Medical Center.

**Christine Dent, R.N., B.S.N., CIC,** is an infection prevention nurse at Saint Alphonsus Regional Medical Center in Boise, ID. She is also a member of the Intermountain Chapter of the American Production and Inventory Control Society.

**Asha Devereaux, M.D., M.P.H.,** is a pulmonary/critical care physician in private practice in Coronado, CA. Dr. Devereaux has 11 years of training and service with the U.S. Navy and formerly served as the ICU director on the Isolation Unit of the USNS Mercy hospital ship. She currently serves as a Steering Committee member for the American College of Chest Physicians Disaster Response Network. She has spearheaded a national conference on disaster preparedness, has published on the topic, and currently serves on the California State Board of the American Lung Association. Dr. Devereaux is also president of the California Thoracic Society and the lead physician advisor of the San Diego Medical Reserve Corps. She received her undergraduate education at the University of California–San Diego followed by her M.D./M.P.H. from Tulane University.

**William Fales, M.D., FACEP,** is an associate professor of emergency medicine at Michigan State University–Kalamazoo Center for Medical Studies. He has been a practicing emergency physician at Kalamazoo's two hospitals since 1993. During this time he has served as the EMS medical director for Kalamazoo County. In 2002 he was appointed regional medical director for healthcare preparedness for the nine counties of southwest Michigan under a federal cooperative agreement with the state of Michigan. Dr. Fales also serves as medical advisor to the Michigan State Police Homeland Security and Emergency Management Division and to the State Police Emergency Support (tactical) Team and Bomb Squads. In these various capacities, he regularly responds to EMS and other public safety incidents locally and throughout Michigan. Dr. Fales chairs the 5th District Medical Response Coalition representing the healthcare, public health, and emergency response communities of southwest Michigan. He is also a member of the 5th District Regional Homeland Security Planning Board. In 2005, Dr. Fales was appointed by the Michigan Department of Community Health to manage the medical needs of hundreds of evacuees from Hurricane Katrina. In 2006, he was asked to serve as the medical advisor to the Federal Joint Operations Center for Superbowl XL in Detroit. Dr. Fales received the Distinguished Service Award from the Michigan Emergency Management Association in 2006. In 2007 he was appointed to the newly established Regional Advisory Council for FEMA Region V (IL, IN, MI, MN, OH, and WI).

He recently became the first physician to complete the Naval Postgraduate School's Homeland Security Executive Leaders Program. A former firefighter and paramedic, Dr. Fales is a graduate of Jefferson Medical College in Philadelphia. He subsequently completed a residency in Emergency Medicine at Geisinger Medical Center in Danville, PA.

**Mary E. Fallat, M.D.,** is professor of surgery at the University of Louisville, division director of pediatric surgery, and chief of surgery at Kosair Children's Hospital in Louisville, KY. She has been actively involved in the care of trauma patients for more than 20 years, with particular interests in pediatric trauma care and prehospital care of the injured patient. Dr. Fallat received an undergraduate degree in biology from Northwestern University and an M.D. from Upstate Medical University in Syracuse, NY. Her surgery residency was at the University of Louisville, with a Pediatric Surgery Fellowship at Children's National Medical Center in Washington, DC. Dr. Fallat participated in the Institute of Medicine project, "The Future of Emergency Care in the U.S. Health System," as a member of the Subcommittee on Pediatric Emergency Care. She is member of the Committee on Trauma of the American College of Surgeons, and recently completed her tenure as the Emergency Services-Prehospital Subcommittee Chair and Executive Committee member. Dr. Fallat has been continuously funded as Principal or Co-Investigator for several Emergency Medical System for Children projects in Kentucky since 1993, and was Principal Investigator for the Trauma-Emergency Medical Services System State Grants to Kentucky in 2001–2006. She served on the Kentucky Board of Emergency Medical Services in 2000–2006. She was instrumental in the process that led Kentucky to achieve trauma system legislation in 2008.

**David A. Fleming, M.D., M.A., FACP,** is professor of medicine and director of the Center for Health Ethics at the University of Missouri School of Medicine, where he has been a faculty member since 1995. He is a former HHS primary care research fellow at the Center for Practical Bioethics at Georgetown University. He practiced internal medicine and geriatrics in North Central Missouri for nearly 20 years prior to his joining Georgetown. Currently he also directs the clinical ethics consult service at University of Missouri Health Care, cochairs the ethics committee, and spends a great deal of time teaching and developing curriculum in health ethics and professionalism in the medical school and other schools at the university. He has also continued his internal medicine practice and teaches in the internal medicine department. His primary areas of research interest include health disparity, care of vulnerable populations, end-of-life care, organizational ethics, and research ethics. Dr. Fleming is also governor for the Missouri Chapter of the American College of Physicians. Dr. Fleming received his B.A. in Zoology, M.A. in Microbiology, and M.D. from the University of Missouri. He also completed an M.A. in Ethics from Georgetown University. Dr. Fleming completed his Internal Medicine residency and chief residency at the University of Missouri in 1980. As director of the MU Center for Health Ethics, he is currently leading a statewide consortium of five ethics centers in Missouri to address the ethical issues of pandemic response. This consortium is developing an ethical framework for planning and responding to pandemic influenza as well as mass casualty events.

**George Foltin, M.D.,** is director of the Center for Pediatric Emergency Medicine at the NYU School of Medicine, where he is an associate professor of pediatrics and emergency medicine. He has also served as director of the Pediatric Emergency Service at Bellevue Hospital since 1987. During his tenure there, he developed the first Pediatric Emergency Medicine Fellowship in the state of New York and has been involved with the education of medical students, residents, fellows, and prehospital providers. He is board certified in Pediatrics, Emergency Medicine, and Pediatric Emergency Medicine. Among his numerous committee activities, he is the chair of the American Academy of Pediatrics District II Committee on Emergency Medical Services for Children, chair of the NYC Task Force on Terrorism Preparedness for Children, and founding president of the New York Society for Pediatric Emergency Medicine. He has published extensively in the field of Emergency Medical Services for Children, and serves as a consultant to the NYC and NYS Departments of Health, as well as to federal programs such as the Maternal and Child Health Bureau and the National Highway Traffic Safety Administration. He recently served on the Institute of Medicine Committee on the Future of Emergency Care in the U.S. Health System and the Pediatric Subcommittee for Future of Health Care.

**Kay Fruhwirth, M.S.N., R.N., MICN,** has more than 25 years of leadership experience in healthcare and emergency management. She is currently an assistant director of the Emergency Medical Services Agency for Los Angeles County, CA, and also serves as the coordinator for the Hospital Preparedness Program for Los Angeles County. She and her staff work with public and private agencies and organizations addressing preparedness and planning activities for the healthcare community.

**Shawn Fultz, M.D., M.P.H.,** joined the Department of Veterans Affairs (VA), Veterans Health Administration (VHA), Office of Public Health and Environmental Hazards (OPHEH) in 2006 as senior medical advisor. Dr. Fultz provides clinical input to the Emergency Management Strategic Healthcare Group and advises the Chief Public Health and Environmental Hazards Officer on areas of public health and emergency management. Prior to joining the OPHEH, he was assistant professor of medicine at Yale University School of Medicine and staff physician at the VA Connecticut Healthcare System. His research career, funded by a VA Health Services Research and Development Career Development Award, focused on HIV infection and comorbid illnesses, including liver injury, hepatitis C, and anemia. He has coauthored more than 16 publications in peer-reviewed journals and over 40 abstracts submitted to scientific meetings. Dr. Fultz completed his undergraduate degree at Pennsylvania State University, and his M.D. at the University of Pittsburgh School of Medicine. His residency in Internal Medicine and a General Medicine Fellowship were both completed at the University of Pittsburgh Medical Center. Dr. Fultz also obtained an M.P.H. in Community and Behavioral Health Sciences from the University of Pittsburgh Graduate School of Public Health.

**Edward Gabriel, M.P.A., AEMT-P,** *see Workshop Planning Committee biosketch.*

**Jim Geiling, M.D.,** is an associate professor of medicine and assistant director of the New England Center for Emergency Preparedness at Dartmouth Medical School. A USUHS graduate, he was a medical corps officer in the Army, retiring in 2003 after a 25-year career. During his career he completed his medical training in internal medicine at Letterman Army Medical Center in San Francisco and later critical care medicine at Walter Reed Army Medical Center. He also studied disaster preparedness and medical response during a one-year fellowship with the HHS Office of Public Health Emergency Preparedness (now ASPR). In 2000 he assumed command of the 200-person medical clinic in the Pentagon, a position where he was called on to use his training in preparedness on September 11, 2001, and later that year during the anthrax attacks. In addition to his Dartmouth appointment, he is also an adjunct assistant professor of military and emergency medicine at USUHS. He has written and spoken extensively in the field of disaster medicine, with recent work focusing on emergency mass critical care. Finally, he is a Fellow in the American College of Physicians, the American College of Chest Physicians (ACCP), and the American College of Critical Care Medicine. He serves the ACCP as chair of its Disaster Network and the Society of Critical Care Medicine as chair of its Fundamentals of Disaster Medicine course.

**Mark Goldstein** was the former EMS coordinator and emergency preparedness coordinator for William Beaumont Hospitals, located in the suburbs of Detroit, for the past 20 years. Recently he relocated to Colorado, where he is the emergency services operations manager at Memorial Health System in Colorado Springs. He has participated with the collaboration efforts for emergency preparedness for mass gatherings such as the All-Star Game, Super Bowl, and World Series in Detroit. He is a member of the ENA Emergency Management and Preparedness Committee and the National Association of EMS Physicians.

**Steven Gravely, M.H.A., J.D.,** is a partner and health care practice group leader at Troutman Sanders LLP in Richmond, VA. Mr. Gravely focuses his practice in the area of health law and disaster preparedness and response issues for critical infrastructure industries. He has represented hospitals and other healthcare providers for more than 20 years in the full spectrum of healthcare legal issues. He serves as special counsel for emergency preparedness and response for the Virginia Office of the Attorney General, and he advises the Health and Medical Subpanel to the Secure Commonwealth Panel on legal aspects of preparedness issues. Mr. Gravely received his J.D. from the University of Richmond, and his M.H.A. from the Medical College of Virginia. Prior to attending law school, Mr. Gravely worked in hospital operations in several health systems. He also has a background as a first responder and several years' experience in fire/EMS.

**LTC(P) Wayne Hachey, D.O., M.P.H.,** *see Workshop Planning Committee biosketch.*

**Dan Hanfling, M.D.,** *see Workshop Planning Committee biosketch.*

**Jack Herrmann, M.S.Ed., N.C.C., L.M.H.C.,** *see Workshop Planning Committee biosketch.*

**John L. Hick, M.D.,** *see Workshop Planning Committee biosketch.*

**James G. Hodge, Jr., J.D., LL.M.,** is the Lincoln Professor of Health Law and Ethics at the Sandra Day O'Connor College of Law and Fellow, Center for the Study of Law, Science, and Technology, at Arizona State University (ASU). He is also a Senior Scholar at the Centers for Law and the Public's Health: A Collaborative at Johns Hopkins and Georgetown Universities and president of the Public Health Law Association. Prior to joining ASU in 2009, he was a professor at the Johns Hopkins Bloomberg School of Public Health; adjunct professor of law at Georgetown University Law Center; executive director of the Centers for Law and the Public's Health; and a core faculty member of the Johns Hopkins Berman Institute of Bioethics. Through his scholarly and applied work, Professor Hodge delves into multiple areas of public health law, global health law, ethics, and human rights. The recipient of the 2006 Henrik L. Blum Award for Excellence in Health Policy from the American Public Health Association, he has drafted (with others) several public health law reform initiatives, including the *Model State Public Health Information Privacy Act*, *Model State Emergency Health Powers Act*, *Turning Point Model State Public Health Act*, and *Uniform Emergency Volunteer Health Practitioners Act*. His diverse, funded projects include work on (1) the legal framework underlying the use of volunteer health professionals during emergencies; (2) the compilation, study, and analysis of state genetics laws and policies as part of a multiyear, NIH-funded project; (3) historical and legal bases underlying school vaccination programs; (4) international tobacco policy for the World Health Organization's Tobacco Free Initiative; (5) legal and ethical distinctions between public health practice and research; (6) legal underpinnings of partner notification and expedited partner therapies; and (7) public health law case studies in multiple states. He is a national expert on public health information privacy law and ethics, having consulted with HHS, CDC, FDA, the Centers for Medicare and Medicaid Services, the Office for Human Research Protections, the American Public Health Association, the Association of Public Health Laboratories, the Council of State and Territorial Epidemiologists and others on privacy issues.

**Rick Hong, M.D., FACEP,** is the medical director for the Public Health Preparedness Section in Delaware's Division of Public Health. He is involved in many statewide emergency preparedness initiatives, such as the Modular Medical Expansion System, In-State Stockpile, and Pandemic Influenza Plan. As chair of Delaware Public Health and Medical Ethics Advisory Group, he is working on incorporating ethics into the prioritization of scarce resources and the development of an altered standard of care. He is also division head of EMS/Disaster Medicine at Cooper University Hospital in Camden, NJ, and practices clinically as an emergency medicine attending physician.

**Robert Hood, Ph.D.,** is the State Public Ethicist at the Florida Department of Health, where he is responsible for the Ethics and Human Research Protection Program. Along with ethics consultation and education about ethical issues in public health practice and research, the program also supports the Department's Institutional Review Boards for review of human subjects research. DOH is the first state health department with a fully accredited human research protection program. He currently chairs the Ethics Subcommittee of the Advisory Committee to the Director of the CDC.

**K. Sue Hoyt, R.N., Ph.D., FNP-BC, CEN, FAEN, FAANP,** is an emergency nurse practitioner at St. Mary Medical Center in Long Beach, CA, and former director of the Master's Entry Program in Nursing at the University of San Diego. Dr. Hoyt is also editor of the *Advanced Emergency Nursing Journal.* She has given more than 100 national and international healthcare-related presentations and has authored nearly 50 publications, including an article titled *The San Diego County Wildfires: Perspectives of Healthcare Providers* in the Journal of Emergency Nursing. Dr. Hoyt is a past president of the ENA and currently the chair of the Advanced Practice Nursing Committee. This committee recently completed a Delphi Study on Competencies for Nurse Practitioners in Emergency Care. Dr. Hoyt is a fellow in both the Academy of Emergency Nursing (FAEN) and the American Academy of Nurse Practitioners (FAANP). She has received numerous honors and awards. Dr. Hoyt was last year's recipient of the AANP State Award for Excellence. She has been a past recipient of ENA's highest distinction, the ENA Lifetime Achievement Award.

**James J. James, M.D., Dr.P.H., M.H.A.,** is director of the American Medical Association's (AMA's) Center for Disaster Medicine and Emergency Response. He manages and develops a comprehensive medical and public health program for AMA's response to terrorism and other disasters. He works with the HHS and state and local medical societies to share information, implement communications strategies, and coordinate medical and public health agencies' responses in the event of a terrorist attack or other sweeping disaster. Dr. James served as director of the Miami-Dade County Health Department from 2000 through 2002. In this role, he was responsible for overseeing public health programs throughout the county, and was instrumental in dealing with the anthrax-related incidents after the September 11, 2001, terrorist attacks. Under Dr. James's leadership, Florida developed a comprehensive plan to respond to future bioterrorist events. He was appointed to Florida Governor Bush's Domestic Security Task Force and as lead health agent for preparedness and response for Region 7, which encompasses the counties of Miami-Dade, Broward, Palm Beach, West Palm Beach, and Monroe. During his tenure, the Miami-Dade Health Department was awarded the 2002 Governor's Sterling Award, which is conferred on businesses and organizations in Florida to acknowledge performance excellence in management and operations. Dr. James served for 26 years with the U.S. Army Medical Department in a variety of roles, including surgeon general (Eight Army, U.S. Forces Korea) and commanding general (William Beaumont Army Medical Center). He is an epidemiologist and is board certified in Preventive Medicine. He holds an M.D. from the Cincinnati College of Medicine and a Dr.P.H. from the University of California–Los Angeles School of Public Health. He also holds a master's degree in Healthcare Administration from Baylor University. In addition, he attended the Armed Forces Staff College and the Industrial College of the Armed Forces.

**Lisa Kaplowitz, M.D., M.S.H.A.,** is the health director for the Alexandria (VA) Health Department, a position she has held since 2008. From 2002 to 2008, she was deputy commissioner for emergency preparedness and response at the Virginia Department of Health (VDH). She was responsible for the development and implementation of Virginia's public health response to all natural and other emergencies. She also coordinated the health department's planning and response with hospitals, the healthcare system, and all state emergency response agencies and organizations in Virginia. She also coordinated Virginia's response with that of adjacent states and the District of Columbia, including the National Capital Region. Before joining VDH, Dr. Kaplowitz was a faculty member in the Department of Medicine at Virginia Commonwealth University (VCU) for 20 years and director of the VCU HIV/AIDS Center. In that role, she developed HIV clinical and training programs and was involved extensively in HIV legislative and policy issues at the state and federal levels. She also was medical director of telemedicine and ambulatory Care for the VCU Health System. She earned her M.D. from the University of Chicago Pritzker School of Medicine, and completed her residency in Internal Medicine and Fellowship in Infectious Diseases at the University of North Carolina–Chapel Hill. She was a Health Policy Fellow with the Institute of Medicine in 1996–97. During her Fellowship, she worked in Senator Jay Rockefeller's office on a number of issues, including Medicare, the State Children's Health Insurance Program, other health financing topics, and end-of-life care. She completed a Master's of Science in Health Administration (M.S.H.A.) at VCU in 2002. In addition to public health and emergency preparedness, she has a strong interest in health policy, healthcare financing, and improving access to health care.

**Kerry Kernen, B.S.N., R.N.,** is the emergency preparedness administrator for Summit County Health District in Ohio. She has practiced as an R.N. for 26 years and has worked in the public health sector for the past 10 years. Within public health she was in the nursing division for 7 years. For the past 3 years, she has focused on emergency preparedness planning, with a major focus on pandemic influenza planning for the past 2½ years. She is currently working on M.S.N.-M.P.A. degrees at Kent State University.

**RADM Ann R. Knebel, R.N., D.N.Sc., FAAN,** *see Workshop Planning Committee biosketch.*

**Kristi L. Koenig, M.D., FACEP,** is an internationally recognized expert in the fields of homeland security, disaster and emergency medicine, emergency management, and emergency medical services. A systems thinker, with a strong academic and health policy background, she is widely published and sought internationally for lectures and presentations. She has been an invited consultant to The Joint Commission, FEMA, the state of California, and the government of Taiwan, among others. A board-certified Emergency Physician, she has been director of public health preparedness for the University of California–Irvine since 2004. In 1999, the Secretary of the VA appointed Dr. Koenig for a 5-year term as national director of the Emergency Management Strategic Healthcare Group and principal advisor on Emergency Management and Disaster Medicine to the Under Secretary for Health where she led emergency management for the nation's largest integrated healthcare system. She concurrently held a position as clinical professor of emergency medicine at The George Washington University School of Medicine and Health Sciences. Prior to joining the VA, Dr. Koenig was director of prehospital and disaster medicine at Highland Hospital in Oakland, CA, and associate professor of emergency medicine at the University of California–San Francisco. In 1996, Dr. Koenig was invited to be codirector of the Accident and Emergency Department at St. George's Hospital National Health Service Trust in London, where she was concurrently director of undergraduate medical student education and Honorary Senior Lecturer at the University of London. An honors graduate in Applied Mathematics from the University of California–San Diego, Dr. Koenig received her M.D. degree from Mount Sinai School of Medicine in New York and completed an Emergency Medicine Residency at Highland Hospital in Oakland, CA, serving as chief resident in her final year. A Fellow of the ACEP, Dr. Koenig is currently professor of emergency medicine and codirector of the EMS and Disaster Medical Sciences Fellowship at the University of California–Irvine School of Medicine.

**Donna Levin, J.D.,** is the general counsel for the Massachusetts Department of Public Health. Prior to her 1988 appointment, Ms. Levin served as a deputy general counsel and concentrated in several different areas of health law, including determination of need, long-term care and hospital regulation, and environmental health. In her current role, she manages the Office of General Counsel and advises the commissioner of public health and senior staff on all legal aspects concerning the implementation of Department responsibilities pursuant to statutory and regulatory authority; major policy initiatives of the Department; and legislation affecting the Department's interests. Most recently, Ms. Levin has focused on the expansion of newborn screening services in the Commonwealth; the review and analysis of the Massachusetts Law on Genetics and Privacy; implementation of the Health Insurance Consumer Protections Law; issues of public health authority and emergency response; and legal oversight of eight professional health boards. Ms. Levin is a member of the Health Law Section Steering Committee of the

Boston Bar Association. She holds a B.A. from the State University of New York at Stony Brook and a J.D. from Northeastern University School of Law.

**CAPT Deborah Levy, Ph.D., M.P.H.,** *see Workshop Planning Committee biosketch.*

**Marianne Lorini, M.B.A.,** has served as the president and CEO of the Akron Regional Hospital Association (ARHA) for the past 11 years. ARHA is an organization focused on facilitating and coordinating services to assist its membership of 19 hospitals in meeting and improving the healthcare needs of the communities in which they serve. ARHA is also responsible for coordinating emergency preparedness activities for 29 acute care hospitals in a 13-county region. Ms. Lorini has over 35 years of hospital experience, including more than 20 years at the Cleveland Clinic Foundation and other hospitals in northeast Ohio. She has also improved hospital operations through her consulting work in Texas, California, and Oregon. Ms. Lorini has a B.S. in Health Services Administration and an M.B.A. from Case Western Reserve University.

**Kevin McCulley** currently serves as the emergency preparedness coordinator and senior data analyst for the Association for Utah Community Health, Utah's association of Community Health Centers (CHCs). He has been involved with the CHC system since 2002, and his work has included disaster preparedness and response, health policy analysis, strategic planning, and community development. In addition, Mr. McCulley serves as a Steering Committee member for the Utah Multicultural Health Network, a lead member of the Utah Health Care Safety Net Summit group, a founder of the Taylorsville Emergency Volunteer Coordinating Committee, a lead member of the Utah Vulnerable Populations Workgroup, and a member and trainer for the South Salt Lake City Community Emergency Response Team. Mr. McCulley has maintained involvement with the Utah Red Cross through the years, from teaching CPR classes to training staff and managing emergency response tents during the 2002 Olympics.

**Margaret (Peggy) M. McMahon, R.N., M.N., CEN,** *see Workshop Planning Committee biosketch.*

**Paula Nickelson** is the special needs population liaison at the Center for Emergency Response and Terrorism in the Missouri Department of Health and Senior Services. In this role, she coordinates emergency planning for special needs populations from a state perspective. Ms. Nickelson's career includes both private and public healthcare management, as well as public health management, with particular emphasis on systems planning and policy development. Her career has afforded multiple opportunities to provide direct services, as well as policy and planning responsibilities for a variety of populations with special needs. Ms. Nickelson serves on Missouri's task force to develop draft altered standards of care.

**J. Patrick O'Neal, M.D.,** is the director of preparedness in the Georgia Division of Public Health. He completed an undergraduate degree in premedicine at Davidson College in North Carolina. Dr. O'Neal received his medical education at the Tulane University School of Medicine. Following medical school, he completed a rotating internship at Providence Hospital, Portland, OR, prior to entering the Air Force for training in flight medicine. Dr. O'Neal served as a flight surgeon in Vietnam in 1970–1971. Upon his return to civilian life, Dr. O'Neal served in Macon, GA, as the director of the Outpatient Clinic at the Medical Center of Central Georgia for 2 years before practicing emergency medicine at Dekalb Medical Center in Decatur, GA. Dr. O'Neal practiced emergency medicine at that facility for 29 years. During his time at Dekalb Medical Center he served as medical director for Dekalb EMS. For his final 7 years at Dekalb Medical Center, he served as the regional medical director for EMS throughout the Greater Atlanta area. Throughout his career in emergency medicine, Dr. O'Neal has been an advocate for trauma system development in Georgia. When he retired as the medical director of the Emergency Department at Dekalb Medical Center in 2002, he became the medical director for the Office of EMS/Trauma in the Georgia Division of Public Health. Currently serving as the preparedness director in the Georgia Division of Public Health, he has oversight responsibility for EMS, trauma, injury prevention, and emergency preparedness.

**Paul R. Patrick** is the director of the Bureau of EMS and Preparedness for the Utah Department of Health. He completed his Design Engineering degree in 1976 from Brigham Young University. Following graduation he worked in the construction industry for 14 years as a supervisor, foreman, and general building contractor. In 1978, he was certified as an

EMT and worked for 25 years as a volunteer with the Springville Ambulance Service. From 1983 to 1986, he served as an affiliate faculty member for the Utah Chapter of the American Heart Association, which he chaired for 2 years. In 1987, he served 2 years on the national faculty for the American Heart Association and currently is a member of the Western Regional Stroke Task Force. In 1988, Mr. Patrick began working for the State of Utah Bureau of Emergency Medical Services as a regional consultant. He received additional training at the state and national levels. In 2000 he became a program manager for the Bureau, supervising the Technical Assistance and Quality Assurance program; in 2005 he also took on the role as acting director for the Bureau. In February 2006, Mr. Patrick was selected as the emergency medical services director and public health and hospital preparedness director for the state of Utah. In April 2006, along with his other duties, he was selected as the deputy director for the Division of Health Systems Improvement for the Utah Department of Health. Mr. Patrick has received many quality awards from the Department of Health. He was involved extensively during the 2002 Salt Lake Winter Olympics, preparations for the 2004 Athens Summer Olympics, and with the many agencies in the state on EMS issues.

**Raymond P. Pepe, J.D.,** is a Pennsylvania delegate to the Uniform Law Commission and a partner in the Harrisburg Office of K&L Gates, an international law firm consisting of more than 1,900 attorneys operating at 32 locations in the United States, Europe, and Asia. His legal practice focuses on matters of administrative law affecting state and local governments, with a strong focus on healthcare issues. In his capacity as a member of the Uniform Law Commission, he served as the chair of the Drafting Committee for the *Uniform Emergency Volunteer Health Practitioner Act* and currently serves as the Commission's Enactment Coordinator for nationwide efforts to promote the adoption of the Uniform Act. Before starting private practice of law, he served as legislative counsel to the Pennsylvania Governor Dick Thornburgh; as chair of the Governor's Task Force for Regulatory Relief; and as counsel to the Pennsylvania House of Representatives. He is a graduate of Georgetown University and Georgetown Law School.

**Cheryl A. Peterson, M.S.N., R.N.,** *see Workshop Planning Committee biosketch.*

**Sally Phillips, Ph.D., R.N.,** (*Workshop Chair*) *see Workshop Planning Committee biosketch.*

**Tia Powell, M.D.,** *see Workshop Planning Committee biosketch.*

**Michael J. Robbins, Pharm.D.,** is the Strategic National Stockpile (SNS) director for the Chicago Department of Public Health. Dr. Robbins is responsible for city planning as it relates to preevent and incident receipt, storage, and distribution of medical materiel in response to public health disasters. Dr. Robbins served as the initial planning pharmacist for the CDC SNS Program. His work included formulary development, response deployments (including 911 and anthrax letters), and initial concept and design of the SNS Chempack Program.

**John T. Robinson, Major USA Ret.,** currently serves as director for safety–security management and emergency preparedness at Baptist Memorial Hospital–North Mississippi (BMH-NM); commander of the North Mississippi State Medical Assistance Team (SMAT); and deputy director of emergency management, Oxford, MS. Mr. Robinson joined the staff of BMH-NM in 1993 as director for safety and security management. He has attended numerous courses on emergency management and has participated in several actual emergency events that occurred in the hospital's service area. The SMAT mentioned above is a 50-bed mobile hospital that can be deployed locally, within the state, or regionally. Mr. Robinson's expertise is in working with local and state government and volunteer organizations to plan for and respond to emergency events.

**Shawn Rogers, EMT-P,** is director of the Emergency Medical Services Division of the Oklahoma State Department of Health. Mr. Rogers completed the EMT basic course at South Oklahoma City Junior College in 1981, and finished the paramedic program the following year. He worked as an EMT intermediate and paramedic at AmCare in Oklahoma City until 1985, when he moved to Yukon EMS. He became the director there in 1986, and started teaching basic and paramedic courses at Moore-Norman Vo-Tech the same year. He was one of the first Prehospital Trauma Life Support (PHTLS) instructors in Oklahoma. Mr. Rogers directed Yukon EMS through its transition into Mercy EMS, and operated that agency from 1987 to 1996. He then joined the Oklahoma State Health Department EMS division, where he served as an EMS administrator and trauma systems coordinator before becoming EMS director in 2001. Mr. Rogers is an executive board member of Advocates for EMS, a national advocacy group, and president-elect of the National Association of State EMS Officials.

**Jeffrey L. Rubin** has been involved in healthcare administration and planning for more than 30 years in both the private and public sectors. His experience includes EMS system development, disaster medical services planning and operations, public health program administration, and primary care clinic management. He currently serves as the chief of the Disaster Medical Services Division of the California Emergency Medical Services Authority. In this capacity he is responsible for the state's policies and plans for the medical response to major disasters and terrorist attacks, and the provision of technical assistance to local governments to enhance their ability to meet the medical needs of victims.

**Catherine Ruhl, C.N.M., M.S.,** is associate director for women's health programs at the Association of Women's Health, Obstetric and Neonatal Nurses (AWHONN) in Washington, DC. She has been a certified nurse midwife for 21 years and currently practices at Providence Hospital in Washington, DC. She obtained her bachelor's degree in Nursing from the University of Kansas and her master's degree in Nursing from the University of Illinois–Chicago. At AWHONN she manages continuing nursing education programs; reviews and contributes content to AWHONN's professional journals; and represents AWHONN to a variety of national organizations, including The Partnership to End Cervical Cancer and the CDC's Select Panel on Preconception Care. She cochaired AWHONN's Emergency Preparedness advisory panel in 2009.

**Floyd K. (Rusty) Russell, Ed.D.,** is a research program coordinator and homeland security liaison in the Office of the Vice President for Research and Economic Development at West Virginia University, reporting to the vice president. He works primarily in the development of homeland security programs, with a focus on interdisciplinary initiatives. He advises the vice president on research and development activities in homeland security, acts as homeland security liaison with external government and industry partners, and develops multidisciplinary projects and funding scenarios with internal and external partners. Current focus areas include community resiliency, energy systems resiliency, public health preparedness and response, and mass population displacement due to high-consequence events. He works with the Resilient Communities Initiative to develop resiliency in rural areas and small cities for catastrophic event mitigation, preparedness, response, and recovery. In previous appointments, he has been a faculty member in the Department of Community Medicine and director of the Virtual Medical Campus. His previous work has focused on understanding the communication and coordination needs of state and local responders to mass disaster events and developing training and knowledge sources for planning and preparedness. He has developed collaborative projects in terrorism and disaster planning and preparedness with funding from DHS and the HHS Health Resources and Services Administration FY03/04 Bioterrorism Curriculum Development and Training Program. Content areas have included hospital emergency management for weapons of mass destruction events, campus security, forensic epidemiology, inclusion of health care in emergency response coordination, and preparedness planning for higher education campus executives.

**Terry L. Schenk** is a consultant for the Florida Department of Health, a certified emergency manager, a former fire chief, and a charter member of the Florida Governor's Domestic Security Oversight Council. He is also a professor of emergency management at St. Petersburg College and wrote Florida's Alternate Care Site Plan. He currently serves as the program manager for prehospital triage, alternative medical treatment sites, and altered care standard planning projects for the Florida Department of Health.

**Valerie Sellers, M.H.A.,** has been with the New Jersey Hospital Association (NJHA) since 1992 and serves as senior vice president of health planning and research. Ms. Sellers oversees activities related to certificate of need, managed care, *Health Insurance Portability and Accountability Act*, community benefit, innovation, emergency preparedness, and other policy and regulatory issues impacting hospitals. She has been responsible for the start-up of three major divisions within NJHA, including Continuing Care, Emergency Preparedness, and NJHA's Institute for Quality and Patient Safety. She is also responsible for research activities related to NJHA's Health Research and Educational Trust. Prior to joining NJHA, Ms. Sellers was the director of administration for 1 of 13 colleges at Cornell University. She graduated from Cornell with an undergraduate degree in Industrial and Labor Relations and a master's degree in Health Administration.

**Cheryl Starling, R.N., M.S.,** *see Workshop Planning Committee biosketch.*

**Leslee Stein-Spencer, R.N., M.S.,** has more than 20 years of experience in planning, organizing, implementing, and managing EMS in a variety of settings. She is a Registered Nurse and currently works for the Chicago Fire Department as manager of quality assurance. She also serves as program advisor to the National Association of State EMS Officials. Ms. Stein-Spencer has represented EMS directors on numerous federal initiatives, including the Interim National Preparedness Goal document, Target Capabilities List, Universal Task List, Interim National Infrastructure Protection Plan, National Incident Management System, and National Response Plan. She also serves as the Principal Investigator in the development of the Model State Emergency Medical Services System document for the nation and Model EMS Legislation. Ms. Stein-Spencer previously worked as a consultant and provided subject-matter expertise on hospital, public health, and emergency medical services system preparedness activities. She has participated in numerous national and international bioterrorism-related discussion panels, and led the development and oversight of bioterrorism initiatives. Ms. Stein-Spencer also served as a team member for the Nationwide Plan Review team for the DHS as well as lead for Public Health and Medical (ESF 8) for the team. Prior to consulting, Ms. Stein-Spencer was chief of the Division of Emergency Medical Services and Highway Safety at the Illinois Department of Public Health for 18 years. During that time, Ms. Stein-Spencer rewrote the EMS Act and rules and regulations; developed and implemented a statewide trauma and facility recognition plan for the pediatrics system; developed and implemented an emergency operation center for the state health department using the principles of Incident Command System (ICS); developed a State Medical Emergency Disaster Plan; and developed and implemented a hospital preparedness assessment tool in which all 187 hospitals responded. Ms. Stein-Spencer also developed and implemented an EMS preparedness assessment tool for EMS providers and EMTs to assess their domestic preparedness and training needs. She coordinated a state medical response to mass casualty incidents and was one of the lead coordinators for TOPOFF 2. Ms. Stein-Spencer was responsible for developing and implementing the Illinois Medical Emergency Response Team and the Illinois Nurse Volunteer Emergency Needs team, which serve as models for the nation. Ms. Stein-Spencer has received numerous awards and recognitions by state and federal agencies.

**Lori A. Upton, R.N., B.S.N., M.S., CEM,** is the assistant director of emergency management for Texas Children's Hospital. Ms. Upton has an extensive background in clinical operations and leadership of EDs and trauma centers and has been involved in emergency management since 1997. Ms. Upton serves on many emergency preparedness planning groups and committees at the local, state, and national levels. She has published several papers on medical responses to disasters and speaks nationally and internationally on this subject. In addition to her role at Texas Children's Hospital, she is also the executive director of the Regional Hospital Preparedness Council. In that capacity she coordinates and prioritizes planning objectives to meet federal preparedness grant requirements and acts as the medical operations chief in the Catastrophic Medical Operations Center for an 18-county region. This coordinated effort was put into action during the response of the Texas Gulf Coast to Hurricanes Katrina, Rita, Gustav, and Ike. She is a certified emergency manager, and holds a bachelor's degree in Nursing from the University of Texas and a master's degree in Emergency Management from Touro University.

**Darlene Weisman, M.S.,** is the regional emergency manager, Region V, for the VHA. She began her career at the VA Medical Center North Chicago as an industrial hygienist, and then served as chief of safety at VA Hines Hospital. Ms. Weisman accepted a position with the VHA's Emergency Management Strategic Healthcare Group as Area Emergency Manager for VISN 12 in 2002. She provided emergency management guidance and oversight to the Veterans Integrated Services Network (VISN) Office and seven VA Hospitals/Medical Centers in three states. She was the Milwaukee Federal Coordinating Center coordinator and designated VA regional liaison for FEMA Region V. She has actively participated in national projects, including the VHA Capabilities Assessment Steering Committee and Presidential Decision Directive 62 Training for NDMS Hospitals Project Advisory Group. She has provided presentations on NDMS definitive care topics at the FEMA Region V Regional Interagency Steering Committee and Milwaukee County Region 7 Board of Directors' meetings. Ms. Weisman had primary responsibility for the development of the Operations Plan for the 2003 Chicago VA Senior Management Conference and was the designated VA representative for TOPOFF 2 in the Chicago area. For these events, she developed written plans that included VISN 12's commitments and involvement, and participated in the exercise and critiques. In 2004, Ms.

Weisman was deployed to VA Miami to assist with recovery efforts from Hurricane Jeanne. She was deployed twice to VAMC Martinsburg to assist with staffing the Emergency Management Strategic Healthcare Group Emergency Operations Center for Hurricanes Katrina and Rita in 2005. While in Martinsburg, she coordinated with the VISN Support Services Center to develop and implement a VHA electronic bed reporting system. Ms. Weisman received the following awards and recognition: TOPOFF 2; 2003 Chicago VA Senior Management Conference; 2005 NDMS Planning Committee, PDD 62; 2004 and 2005 hurricane relief efforts; and the Incident Response Communication Team support for the 2008 Republican National Convention. She received a B.S. and M.S. from Michigan State University.

**Tim Wiedrich, M.B.A.,** is the emergency preparedness and response section chief at the North Dakota Department of Health, and he also directs the department's Division of Education Technology. Mr. Wiedrich joined the Department of Health in 1984 as a program representative for the Division of Emergency Medical Services and was appointed director in 1988. He received bachelor's and master's degrees in Business Administration and Management from the University of Mary, as well as a public health certificate in preparedness, response, and recovery from the University of Minnesota. Before joining the state health department, Mr. Wiedrich served as chief investigator for the North Dakota Attorney General's Consumer Fraud and Antitrust Division. He was also a volunteer for the Beulah, ND, ambulance service for 10 years.

**Deb Wynkoop, M.P.A.,** is currently the director of health policy at the Utah Hospitals and Health Systems Association, where she is responsible for the operation and support of the Association's health policy initiatives, including overview of all Utah Department of Health, Commerce, and Human Service programs and regulatory matters as they relate to the hospital community. Ms. Wynkoop has a B.S. in Recreational Therapy and an M.P.A. Previously she worked for the state of Utah for 27 years. Her last appointment was as director of the Bureau of Licensing, Utah Department of Health, where she was responsible for licensing and regulating healthcare facilities statewide. She has extensive experience in public health, administrative rule processes, and the legislative process. Ms. Wynkoop is a Fellow in the American Association for Intellectual and Developmental Disabilities.